ON IVF

(IN VITRO FERTILIZATION)

THE *Dignity* SERIES

ON IVF
(IN VITRO FERTILIZATION)

STEPHANIE GRAY CONNORS

WORD on FIRE

Published by Word on Fire, Elk Grove Village, IL 60007

Printed in Italy

Cover design and interior art direction by Nicolas Fredrickson;
typesetting by Marlene Burrell

While all stories in this book are true, some names and identifying information
have been changed to protect the privacy of the individuals involved

ISBN: 978-1-68578-249-8

Library of Congress Control Number: 2024945110

To my sister Mary: Your outpouring of wisdom has guided and blessed me through many years of ministry. It is you I have to thank for convincing me to write this book when I did.

Contents

Series Introduction

Why dignity? Because human dignity (*dignitas*, the worthiness of each person) is the foundation of all human society. Jacques Maritain, the Catholic philosopher who helped draft the United Nations Universal Declaration of Human Rights, affirmed this in saying, "The privilege connected with the dignity of the person is inalienable, and human life involves a sacred right."

In a time of political polarization, social division, and the ongoing "culture wars," the Dignity Series aims to refocus our attention on human dignity. The series enters into the great mystery of human life with wonder and reverence, and unflinchingly faces grave threats to human dignity, many of them ignored in the culture today.

Each volume in the series will examine one of those threats, drawing on rational argument, spiritual sources, and above all, personal stories that take readers into the lived experience on the frontier of the issue. This broad mix of ideas and approaches acknowledges that a wide variety of backgrounds and personalities shape how we interact with these questions—and that if a book is to help us grow, it has to stir our hearts as well as activate our minds.

The Dignity Series emerges out of and points back to the whole-life ethic of Catholic social teaching, which is grounded in the principle of human dignity. "Social justice," the *Catechism of the Catholic Church* teaches, "can be obtained only in respecting the transcendent dignity of man" (*CCC* 1929). And that dignity, on the Catholic reading, can only finally rest on our status as creatures made in the image and likeness of God (Gen. 1:26). However, these books are for anyone—Catholic or non-Catholic, religious or non-religious—who wrestles with these issues and longs to see a more informed and considerate approach to them.

To see a full list of titles in the Dignity Series, please visit wordonfire.org/dignity.

Introduction

"Do you have any siblings?"
"Yes, I do."
"How many?"
"Well, if you count half-siblings, I have five hundred to a thousand."

While the numbers in that imaginary dialogue may sound like a joke, they are not—thanks to modern reproductive technologies. In the documentary *Anonymous Father's Day*, viewers meet the man behind this story. His biological father was a sperm donor, and hundreds of humans are his father's offspring—and thus his brothers and sisters—as a result.

Or consider the Donor Sibling Registry website. It was created in the year 2000 to connect people who are genetically related to one another as a result of others who gave away their sperm, eggs, or embryos. The largest group the website has brought together so far is two hundred half-siblings. One sperm donor linked up through that registry donated four hundred times in his lifetime, and since one donation can produce twenty-four vials, the fertility clinics he worked with could have sold as many as 9,600 vials. It is therefore within the realm of possibility that this donor fathered hundreds, if not thousands, of biological children around the world. Currently, he is aware of twenty-two.

Stories like these raise this important question: Is it ethical to create human beings by science and not by sex?

In vitro fertilization (IVF) is one such procedure that makes children by way of science. With IVF, sperm and eggs are harvested from a man and a woman, combined in a petri dish where fertilization occurs, and the resulting human embryos begin their lives in glass ("in vitro") instead of in their mother's body. Ultimately, at least one, if not more, of the embryos will be transferred into a woman's body.

Sometimes the sperm and eggs are the gametes of a husband and wife who are having difficulty conceiving naturally and enlist the help of science to establish fertilization in a lab. Other times, sperm and/or eggs are provided by third parties that are not the couple planning to parent. In some cases, the sperm is from one partner of a gay couple, but eggs are provided by a woman. Sometimes—and certainly this is the case with the latter scenario—surrogacy is pursued, where a woman is contracted to gestate a child in her womb and then relinquish the child at birth to the individual or couple who commissioned the baby's production.

Should IVF be embraced or rejected? Is it inherently good or inherently evil? Or, perhaps, is it something that is sometimes right and other times wrong, depending on the circumstances?

These are important questions to consider, because IVF is now widespread and international, affecting millions upon millions of people. Celebrities are increasingly divulging their infertility struggles and pursuit of IVF, including the Obamas, Nicole Kidman, and Céline Dion. These aren't isolated cases. In 2018, CNN reported that since 1978, when Louise Brown became the first successful "test tube baby," there have been a minimum of eight million children born around the world who were conceived through IVF and related technology. That number is only climbing, with estimates showing that more than five hundred thousand babies are born annually around the world as a result of IVF.

For every one embryo that successfully matures to birth, typically several others are created—sometimes ten or more embryos. IVF-conceived persons are in our families, churches, workplaces, and the general public. So are the people who attempted IVF, whether they were successful or not. We are talking about tens of millions of human beings, at a minimum, who are directly impacted by this technology in some way.

And the impact is not only on individuals; it is also on society as a whole, and it spills over into public policy. That became abundantly clear in 2024 when the Alabama Supreme Court came out with a ruling related to IVF that caused an uproar and led to debate across the United States. The case under consideration involved couples who sued their fertility clinic because their frozen embryos had been destroyed by a hospital patient who wandered into the room where their embryos were in the freezer. The patient removed them and dropped them, leading to the demise of the embryos.

The court ruled that embryos not within a womb were to be considered children under the law; in other words, Alabama's Wrongful Death of a Minor Act applied to all preborn children, including the youngest of our kind: newly conceived embryos not yet inserted in a woman's body. A justice wrote, "Unborn children are 'children' under the Act, without exception based on developmental stage, physical location, or any other ancillary characteristics."

In response, IVF clinics in the state were hesitant to continue operating for fear of legal ramifications. Patients with scheduled appointments were devastated, many publicly sharing their stories of struggling with infertility, being on the cusp of an embryo transfer attempt, and being left in limbo about whether they would be able to access IVF in their state going forward.

Rallies and protests were held. Media coverage was extensive. Public figures on both sides weighed in as a national debate erupted. And Alabama legislators were quick to respond, passing a bill "to provide civil and criminal *immunity* for death or damage to an embryo to any individual or entity when providing or receiving services related to in vitro fertilization." Even at a federal level, Senator Ted Cruz put forward legislation called the IVF Protection Act, which went so far as to propose that states that ban IVF access be denied Medicaid funding.

In light of such intense political and personal debate, this book aims to ethically evaluate the increasingly common practice of IVF, presenting arguments that are both sectarian and nonsectarian in nature. Although explicitly Christian appeals are made, a variety of information is offered to provoke deep thought and consideration, even for those who embrace a different religion or no religion at all. If we were to view the sections of this book like a house, part 1 lays the foundation with basic principles and ideas to guide our overall thinking on the topic; part 2 looks at the effects of IVF and identifies walls that should be in place; and part 3 is all about design: it proposes a blueprint for how to view sexuality, reproductive technologies, and life itself in this broken world. More than just an examination of IVF's morality, this book shares stories of people who have endured the great suffering of infertility and offers a variety of hope-filled responses.

It also includes my own story. While some people have difficulty *getting* pregnant, in my case I've had difficulty *sustaining* pregnancies. In my first three years of marriage, I had four miscarriages, three of which were in a row. Never getting to cradle in my arms children I so desperately wanted was devastating. Losing child after child made me question whether I could emotionally handle getting pregnant again; even though I wanted more children, I feared more losses. Recurrent miscarriage is often listed as a reason to pursue IVF.

So is age. I didn't begin trying to have children until I was forty, the age when the likelihood of pregnancy drops to a mere 5 percent each menstrual cycle. Even though my body has an unusual ability to defy the odds in that regard, my experience of many miscarriages aligns with another negative aspect of my age: miscarriage risk climbs to roughly 40 percent at age forty. My husband and I chose not to pursue IVF, although we were helped with the aid of Restorative Reproductive Medicine, explained in chapter 12.

Experiencing unmet desire, living through loss, finding hope in alternatives, and surrendering to a power higher than my own—all these helped form my perspective through difficult times, which I hope will help others as well.

PART I
Laying the Foundation

1

The Pain Is Real

When a person longs for something that is good, something they are made for, then to not have that desire fulfilled is an experience of profound suffering and anguish. I think, for example, of a documentary I watched several years ago about men in China who were searching for wives but were not able to find a life partner. Due to a culture that embraced a one-child policy for more than thirty years, as well as Chinese society's preference for male children, countless baby girls were killed by abortion and infanticide over multiple decades. Years later, when the peers of those missing girls—lots and lots of boys—grew up, they faced a profound gender imbalance. In fact, numbers show that there are thirty-four million *more* men than women in China.

That number is almost the same as the entire population in my birth country of Canada. It is astounding to imagine every single person north of the forty-ninth parallel being male. This comparison helps put into perspective that we are talking about a massive number of human beings who will statistically never find the wife they are longing for.

News station France 24 aired a story about the devastating effects of this gender imbalance. They interviewed a thirty-four-year-old man who lives in a rural village and who has been unable to find a wife. Listening to him speak about this reality is deeply painful. I felt profound empathy for this man in his suffering. He shared his embarrassment of still being single when his peers married ten years earlier. He said, "Not having found a wife yet, I feel my heart is empty." He continued, "I feel like I'm invisible."

His is not an isolated experience. There are millions upon millions more men like him in China. Whether they feel inadequate, lonely, or like a failure, their pain is real. One can find story after story of single men who are living life with dead spirits, constantly feeling dejected and purposeless, and it's enough to make you weep.

The desire for a life companion is similar to the desire for a child: It is good. It is natural. It is ordered. It is what most of us were made for. And just as the unfulfilled desire for a spouse hurts, so does the unfulfilled desire for a child. It hurts a lot.

One of my friends faced infertility for the first four years of her marriage. She said, "The hardest was hearing about abortion. For this I was frustrated with God. Why would he give babies to women that did not want them but would not give me a baby after I had been so careful to do everything in my power to be able to have a baby?" She also shared the monthly sorrow and disappointment she experienced upon the arrival of her period—a vivid reminder that infertility would, cycle after cycle, continue to be her story: "That day was really rough," she said.

Eventually, my friend and her husband adopted as well as managed to conceive, but then they went through an inexplicable year and a half of four miscarriages. Of that cross she explained,

> The worst one physically and emotionally was my second one that ended in me passing out in the bathtub, covered in my own blood and having to go to the hospital in the ambulance for a D&C [dilation and curettage]. This one also introduced me to the life of grey: After this miscarriage, the world was grey and everything felt hard to do. Getting out of bed felt like climbing a large mountain. Laundry, cooking, spending time with my kids . . . the joy had been sucked out of my life. This persisted for multiple months until I spoke to a friend about it and she shared a similar experience after her miscarriage. For some reason just saying it out loud and having these feelings validated really helped.

Another friend of mine told me that her longing for a baby was so deep that seeing her friends get pregnant amplified her own pain. She mentioned not even going to a baby shower for one of her friends because it was too strong of a reminder of what she was lacking. My friend Lea (whose story is told in chapter 12) went through similar emotions when she struggled between wanting to be joyful for a friend's pregnancy announcement and feeling the sting of not yet having her own desire fulfilled. Just recalling the encounter for my interview convicted her that she had covetousness to repent of, but her point was to convey the raw and overpowering emotion that can come with unmet desire.

It took my friends Sadie and Bryan a year to conceive their first child. Then they went six years before conceiving their second. This is referred to as secondary infertility. Sadie found some comments from people would really hurt. For example, she felt frustrated when friends would speak so nonchalantly, even jokingly, about their husbands getting vasectomies after being given precious babies, when she and her husband yearned to have more children so badly. She also shared that it was stressful to be around extended family when they would look at Sadie and Bryan's son and say, "Only one?" Then there were awkward situations where Sadie would not want to go to events where she would run into people she hadn't seen in a while, because she knew they would be expecting her to have more children.

My friend Tessa burst into tears when an elderly lady at church approached her and her husband and said, "When are you going to have children?" Little did she know the deep longing in their hearts that was unfulfilled month after month, and how the question felt like a knife cutting through her heart.

My friends Mariam and Kenneth went into marriage knowing conception would be difficult, if not impossible (the latter was, indeed, to become their story). Mariam was twenty-two when they tied the knot and had never had a period. Only after marriage did she go through serious medical investigations and learned her body had not completed puberty. She went through years of hormone treatments and all kinds of concoctions of drugs to both mature her body physiologically as well as to try to help them conceive. Mariam described this as a roller coaster, and after years of physical and emotional toll, they stopped the interventions, which they had determined to be futile.

My friends Claire and Jeremiah also went into marriage knowing they might have problems conceiving. Claire noticed strange patterns in her cycle that caused her to see a doctor before getting married. A couple weeks after their wedding, they went to an ob-gyn who was a specialist in the Creighton model of fertility treatment (see chapter 12). The news was not good: Claire was told she had polycystic ovary syndrome (PCOS), insulin resistance (making her prediabetic), low progesterone, and hypothyroidism. She was told that she was probably not ovulating. For someone who was only twenty-two years old and had not had health problems before, this was entirely overwhelming, especially as a newlywed. Claire described herself as feeling "broken." The first year and a half of their marriage was very difficult; it felt like a dark cloud was hanging over them. There were so many doctor appointments and so many drug cocktails that required various times of fasting as well as consumption, and it was a headache to keep track of it all. Jeremiah said that there was a lot of tension and stress. Claire talked about the cross of infertility being so heavy. She didn't even want to make friends with a new woman who had moved to town because that woman got pregnant right away—with twins. Claire described how she was constantly looking for information about infertility and what they could do; it became all-consuming and overwhelming.

And then there are my friends Maddy and Peter. They began intentionally trying to get pregnant during the summer of 2018. For the next five years, they lived with the grief of miscarrying the one child they conceived and with monthly reminders of not getting pregnant again. They described this as "heartbreak" and "feeling like a failure." Maddy was diagnosed as having between stage 3 and stage 4 (of 4 stages) endometriosis, which even spread to her diaphragm. Living in Canada, she was on a very long wait list just to see a specialist surgeon who could address the problem; then there was another wait list after that for actually scheduling surgery. They lived through much emotional turmoil (as well as physical turmoil for Maddy, who had excruciatingly painful periods due to the endometriosis). Mother's Day was particularly hard for Maddy. Each year at church, mothers are invited to stand up; she expressed being torn about doing so because although she is a mother to their little one in heaven, she knew she would face comments from observers like, "You're pregnant? When are you due?" One Mother's Day after her miscarriage, her brother-in-law brought flowers to all the female relatives who had children. Maddy was overlooked, and although her brother-in-law did not intend to hurt her, disregarding that she was a mother (albeit to a deceased child) stung her deeply.

Various people have said insensitive things without realizing her private pain. One colleague said, "The clock is ticking, Maddy; time to get going." People observed the timeline since she was married and expected her to have a baby. Someone who did happen to know about her miscarriage made minimizing comments: "At least your miscarriage was early on; at least you didn't have a stillbirth." There is no denying the brutal suffering that comes from losing a child at birth; however, one can also suffer profoundly when losing a child earlier. Maddy said, "When people talk about infertility and miscarriage flippantly as though it's not a big deal, it's hard for me because it's the biggest cross in my life."

2

That Hurts Too!

As the previous stories reveal, the pain of infertility is very real. Sometimes it runs so deep that those experiencing it are not ready to have an intellectual or ethical conversation about how to respond. They do not want to listen to someone lecture them about what they should or should not do, what is right or wrong; they just want someone to sit with them and acknowledge their pain.

I remember a time when I was going through a difficult season emotionally and shared with a friend about what was weighing on me. After laying open my heart to her, she asked me, "What would be most helpful for you right now? Do you want me to tell you what I think or do you want me to just sit in the pain with you?"

Affirmation and validation are very powerful. We feel heard when someone says, "I'm sorry. You're right: it feels unfair and it's a terribly heavy cross. I don't know why this is happening." And there absolutely is a time for that.

To be fully human, it is important to remember that we have both hearts and minds. We can, and should, *feel* deeply, but we are also made with a rational nature. We are designed to *think* deeply too. So there is a time to just sit in the pain. And then there is a time to wrestle with it. But wrestling hurts.

For someone who is in a place where they want validation about their legitimate agony of infertility, they might just want to pause for a bit after reading the previous chapter, with the stories of people who have walked that road before. And yet there comes a time for them to eventually turn the page, which brings us here.

When using our rational nature to think deeply about a moral issue, we might experience a new kind of pain. Instead of pain from an unmet desire, it is the pain that comes from things like critique, judgment, disappointment, or guilt.

In Paul's Second Letter to the Corinthians, he speaks of writing a letter of rebuke and criticism and how the people initially responded to it with distress. He says, "For even if I made you sorry with my letter, I do not regret it (though I did regret it, for I see that I grieved you with that letter, though only briefly). Now I rejoice, not because you were grieved, but because your grief led to repentance; for you felt a godly grief, so that you were not harmed in any way by us. For godly grief produces a repentance that leads to salvation and brings no regret" (2 Cor. 7:8–10).

When someone makes a moral criticism about another's behavior, it can sometimes be received as a personal attack. This is why people of goodwill who wish to grow in virtue should strive to handle such moments with great discipline. Instead of giving way to hurt feelings, we should step back and honestly consider whether there is merit to our critic's view. If there isn't, we could benefit from this thoughtful approach by becoming more convinced of our position. But if there is merit to the criticism, we will benefit from this thoughtful approach by embracing the opportunity to learn and to change our behavior, doing better in our future than in our past.

Criticism can be a momentous occasion for growth. Look at the business world: The best businesses prioritize critiques and evaluation. They are constantly asking what they did wrong and how they can improve. The ones that succeed are the ones that are not afraid to change course when facts and reason disprove what seemed to be good ideas.

In Paul's Second Letter to Timothy, he writes about some people seeking out messengers who tickle their ears with what they want to hear, noting that Timothy, and we, have a responsibility to be faithful to our duty of proclaiming truth, remembering that it is the truth that will make us free (see John 8:32):

> In the presence of God and of Christ Jesus, who is to judge the living and the dead, and in view of his appearing and his kingdom, I solemnly urge you: proclaim the message; be persistent whether the time is favorable or unfavorable; convince, rebuke, and encourage, with the utmost patience in teaching. For the time is coming when people will not put up with sound doctrine, but having itching ears, they will accumulate for themselves teachers to suit their own desires, and will turn away from listening to the truth and wander away to myths. As for you, always be sober, endure suffering, do the work of an evangelist, carry out your ministry fully. (2 Tim. 4:1–5)

Some of the ideas I propose in this book may be challenging. They might hurt to hear. And yet I feel a great responsibility to provide sound ideas, trusting that, deep down, we all experience freedom when we embrace truth over myth. I think we all know that there is something worse than being wrong: it is being wrong *and* not admitting it. Author Matthew Kelly once reflected,

> I have constantly asked myself: *What do I respect?* And at a deep level, I think there is only one thing I truly and deeply respect over and over again in time, and that is virtue. I respect virtue. Virtue inspires me. Virtue in other people challenges me. Virtue raises me up. Virtue allows me to catch a glimpse of what is possible. Virtue gives me hope for the future of humanity. . . .
>
> Our culture has reduced all virtue to the universal virtue of niceness, which is no virtue at all. People comment, "Oh, she is such a nice woman" or "He is such a nice man," which in essence very often means that this man or woman never says or does anything to upset the person making the comment, never ruffles any feathers, never challenges anyone to rise to greater virtue. . . . I hope nobody who knows me ever describes me as "nice" in this context. I hope to upset the people around me occasionally, to rattle them from time to time, to challenge them in ways that make them feel uneasy. . . .
>
> Love makes demands upon us. To love someone means that from time to time you will be required by that love to tell someone something that they would rather not hear.

Thomas Aquinas defined love as willing the other's good. And so it is from that place that the following ideas are proposed.

3

Means vs. Ends and How vs. Who

Let's return to chapter 1's reference to the gender imbalance in China. As terrible as so many men's suffering is there, it has led to a very ugly byproduct: human trafficking. The France 24 news story revealed the alarming practice of women (single or married) being kidnapped and forced into marriages. There simply are not enough women to match the number of men, and some people are responding to this with desperate measures, treating women as property, trafficking them as modern-day slaves, forcing them into relationships they do not want.

The *Washington Post* shared a horrifying story of a Cambodian woman who went to China due to the promise of a job. But when she arrived, she was forced into a marriage against her will. She reported, "My husband said to me: 'You are my slave; I bought you. If I want, I can do anything to you.'" And anything he did: he demanded to have sex four times per day, he beat her after she refused sex when she had given birth only seven days earlier, and his family locked her in the home.

Even when some trafficked marriages do not appear to be as brutal as that, being in a "better" situation does not make it right. For example, the thirty-four-year-old quoted in chapter 1 who was miserable because he was single, a bachelor named Jing Lansui, finally left his village to go in search of a wife in Indonesia. He found one in a woman named Lai, but as France 24 reported, "Lansui paid her smugglers 10,000 euros. Part of that sum was given to Lai's father in exchange for his daughter's hand in marriage." She only knew a few words in Mandarin and certainly not the dialect in her husband's village where she'd be living. Watching video footage of Lansui's parents and other villagers gather around Lai to stare at her like she's an exotic animal as she nervously sits in a foreign atmosphere is truly heartbreaking.

There is no denying the understandable desire for an exclusive relationship with a lifelong partner. The above, however, demonstrates a foundational ethical principle: the end doesn't justify the means. In other words, the very wonderful "end" of marriage doesn't justify the evil "means" of trafficking. No matter how legitimate and good our desires are, these do not give a person license to fulfill the desire *by any means possible*—enslavement (even by a "kind owner") being an obvious example.

Understanding this principle through forced marriage in China helps give insight into the morality of becoming a parent. The same principle of the end not justifying the means applies here. The good end of becoming a parent is not justified when an immoral means is used. For example, it would not be ethical to become a parent by kidnapping a newborn from a hospital. Through this example, we can see that the desire for children does not give a couple license to fulfill their longing by *any* means technically possible. Although the immorality of kidnapping as a means to achieve parenthood is clear to almost everyone, less obvious to many is the immorality of IVF as a means to achieve parenthood. Could it be wrong?

Considering that question is challenging because IVF is how some people have come into existence. That means examining the possibility of it being immoral seems to call into question the value of the people conceived that way.

Some of us were conceived on our parents' blissful honeymoon. Others were a result of a one-night stand. Still others, like my friend Ryan, came to be through the brutality of rape. And due to technology, others have come into existence through IVF. In looking at these four circumstances, we can rightly conclude that they are not equal. A one-night stand based on using another person for sexual pleasure has nothing on the beauty of permanent love grounded in a marital vow of lifelong commitment through "good times and bad." And rape is far more horrifying than a one-night stand, however flawed the latter might also be compared to a loving marriage.

Although the circumstances under which someone comes into being may be good or bad, ideal or not, the greatness of *who* comes to be is independent of all that. Each human is equal in dignity to all others regardless of how we are conceived, and each of us is unrepeatable and irreplaceable. A human person's dignity is inherent to her being, which means that the moment she begins to exist is the moment she has dignity. Science teaches that beings that reproduce sexually (for example, dogs, cats, *and* humans) begin their lives at fertilization. That is a point that would take us beyond the scope of this book and that I unpack in other writings, so I won't go into detail on that here. But it is worth pointing out that the positive contribution of IVF to our world is that it has reinforced that life begins at fertilization. An IVF specialist is not satisfied with a sperm sample alone or with just the harvesting of eggs. The moment an IVF specialist is trying to achieve in the lab is the moment of fertilization, because it is then that we have a genetically new individual who is the next generation, the biological offspring of the parents. After fertilization, the preborn child grows and develops, just as after birth a newborn child grows and develops. *How* we look as adults today and *what* we know intellectually are dramatically different from when we were ten years old, five years old, a newborn, a fetus, or an embryo. But *who* we are as adults today is the same throughout the duration of our lives, beginning at conception.

Because our dignity is grounded in who we are, that means that *how* we were conceived has no bearing on our worth. In other words, among a group of four humans, if one is conceived as a result of marital love, another from lust, a third via violence, and a fourth through technology, while the circumstances or "means" of these conceptions are not all equal or good, the "end" (i.e., each resulting human being) is.

People should rest assured, then, that any moral criticism of IVF does not, and must not, call into question the worth of the child conceived. All humans bear the image of God and should be treated as such, regardless of the circumstances under which they came to be.

4

Rights and Gifts

There is a lot of talk in our world about rights. People will defend a right to life, a right to free speech, a right to own property, and so forth. To have a right to something means you have a just claim to it. You're entitled to it. You can demand it.

Do we have a right to demand a child?

A child is a person. A child is a subject and not an object, and we cannot lay claim to the former as we do to the latter. Why is slavery wrong? Because it involves possessing another. It denies a fundamental principle of civil societies: human beings are equal. If we say we may own another, or have a right to another, then we are creating a situation where we raise ourselves *above* the other. No longer, then, do we have equality, but instead we introduce the dynamic of superiority versus inferiority.

Some might respond to this claim by bringing up parental rights. Doesn't that indicate rights over a child? Perhaps, but not in the way one has a right over property. When we speak of parental rights, we are referring to protecting the child from other parties, such as strangers, and making decisions for the child when the child is incapable of making decisions for herself. As long as a child is not sufficiently mature to act as an independent adult, then someone older, who is charged with the responsibility of caring for the well-being of the child, needs to do that. Because parents, by nature, are designed to love and care for their offspring and do so in a profoundly sacrificial way that we typically do not do for other people, it is parents who are best suited to make decisions *in the best interests of their child*. Parental rights are oriented, ultimately, to the good of the child.

Consider it this way: If someone breaks into your home and steals something that you have purchased with your hard-earned money, you have a right to seek retribution. Your property was unjustly taken. But what if someone breaks into your home and kidnaps your child? You have a right to seek retribution not because your "property" was taken but because the child was harmed. The child has a right to life and to the loving environment of her parents. Kidnapping the child is, first and foremost, an injustice *to the child*, whereas stealing property is, first and foremost, an injustice to you.

If we do not have a right to a fellow human, how should we view each other? A child, like any human, should be viewed as an image-bearer, as someone to love and be loved by, as a gift. A gift is a blessing; it is something bestowed generously and freely from one party to another and given because the giver expects the receiver to be delighted and filled with joy. A gift can only rightly be given by the person who originally possesses the gift. If one human may not possess another, then who possesses a human?

Our Creator, God, does. As Jeremiah 1:5 declares, "Before I formed you in the womb I knew you." Who is the "I" in that passage? It is "the LORD" (Jer. 1:4). Consider these passages from the Psalms:

> O Lord, *you* have searched me and known me.
> *You* know when I sit down and when I rise up;
> *you* discern my thoughts from far away.
> *You* search out my path and my lying down,
> and are acquainted with all my ways.
> Even before a word is on my tongue,
> O Lord, *you* know it completely.
> *You* hem me in, behind and before,
> and lay *your* hand upon me.
> Such knowledge is too wonderful for me;
> it is so high that I cannot attain it. . . .
> For it was *you* who formed my inward parts;
> *you* knit me together in my mother's womb.
> I praise *you*, for I am fearfully and wonderfully made.
> Wonderful are *your* works;
> that I know very well.
> My frame was not hidden from *you*,
> when I was being made in secret,
> intricately woven in the depths of the earth.
> *Your* eyes beheld my unformed substance.
> In *your* book were written
> all the days that were formed for me,
> when none of them as yet existed. (Ps. 139:1–6, 13–16;
> emphasis added)

Consider the story of an American woman named Stephanie Levesque. She was a surrogate on several occasions. The third time, when she was sixteen weeks pregnant, physicians discovered that the child she was carrying had heart problems. The biological parents who had enlisted her surrogacy wanted her to abort the child as a result. She refused and carried the pregnancy to term. In a news story, she expressed grief over how she was cut off from information about the child's status; she doesn't know how he's doing or if he's even still alive. This very negative surrogacy experience, however, did not change her support of surrogacy in general. Rather than work against the practice going forward, she is working to change the parameters and contracts surrounding it. (This is still morally problematic and is addressed later in the book.) She spoke very positively about her previous two surrogacies, and here's what is striking as it pertains to the theme of this chapter: when describing surrogacy, she says, "It is *the* most beautiful gift you could ever give." Then at the end of the news story, the reporter adds, "So she's writing a book about joy—the joy of giving families a baby they never thought they'd have."

Here is a vital question: Although she views her surrogacy as gift-giving, and therefore has good motives and not malicious intentions, *is it her gift to give?*

Imagine, for example, you noticed a child looking longingly at a toy in a store. Then imagine you overheard the parents tell the child he could not have it because the family was too poor to make the purchase. I imagine your heart would break for the child. You would grieve at his disappointment. Now imagine you wanted to make the child experience surprise, joy, and delight, so you gifted the toy to him as he walked out of the store. But imagine you did not purchase the toy for him; imagine you stole it. We all know intuitively that as much as the child would be delighted by the gift, since it was not yours to give, you actually did not have the right to give it.

Although no analogy is perfect, this one does help us to gain insight into the issue of surrogacy and reproductive technologies as a whole. Too easily, well-meaning people can mistakenly fall into the trap of viewing the creation and sustaining of life for a couple who cannot achieve it themselves to be a gift they give to the couple. But we may not give the gift of life when we ourselves do not possess it.

Someone might object as follows: "God could work through others to give his gift of life. We use our intellect all the time to create medicine and other interventions to benefit the human condition. Couldn't IVF and surrogacy be viewed along those lines? Couldn't these be seen as working with God the Creator to respond to the brokenness that exists in this imperfect world?"

That is a good question. God certainly works through others to heal and restore. Just consider this story from the Scriptures:

> One day Peter and John were going up to the temple at the hour of prayer, at three o'clock in the afternoon. And a man lame from birth was being carried in. People would lay him daily at the gate of the temple called the Beautiful Gate so that he could ask for alms from those entering the temple. When he saw Peter and John about to go into the temple, he asked them for alms. Peter looked intently at him, as did John, and said, "Look at us." And he fixed his attention on them, expecting to receive something from them. But Peter said, "I have no silver or gold, but what I have I give you; in the name of Jesus Christ of Nazareth, stand up and walk." And he took him by the right hand and raised him up; and immediately his feet and ankles were made strong. Jumping up, he stood and began to walk, and he entered the temple with them, walking and leaping and

> praising God. All the people saw him walking and praising God, and they recognized him as the one who used to sit and ask for alms at the Beautiful Gate of the temple; and they were filled with wonder and amazement at what had happened to him. (Acts 3:1–10)

Here we see Peter acknowledging Jesus being the power through which the man was healed, but God still used the Apostle as an instrument. Similarly, some might argue that God could work his healing power through the instrument of science to correct that which has gone wrong in nature. And yet, it is important to consider that even when science is enlisted to heal, there are always parameters. For example, it is not ethical to do medical experiments without informed consent. It is not right to use one's surgical skill to transplant an organ for one person that was stolen from another. Or if a pregnant woman experiences nausea, it is not moral to give her the drug thalidomide to relieve her suffering since that pharmaceutical has been found to cause serious congenital malformations.

So what parameters should be set around the creation and sustaining of new life—a life that we can agree may not be owned and is not our gift to give? That requires a deep dive. Before unpacking that fully, let's start by examining more obvious concerns about IVF.

PART 2
Building Walls

5

Harming Preborn Humans

With IVF, it is common practice to create more embryos than initially (if ever) will be implanted in a woman. This is because one cannot be guaranteed that placing an embryo in a woman will lead to the child implanting and growing until birth. To increase the chances of ultimately having a successful pregnancy, many embryos are typically made. A fertility clinic in Kansas described it this way: "Most couples have at least three to five or more embryos frozen to increase their chances of IVF success and/or to use for future IVF cycles when they are ready for Baby #2, 3, or 4."

Take, for example, a couple who used social media to share their IVF journey. They posted a video on YouTube titled "Fertilization Report." They announced that the wife had had thirty-one eggs retrieved (which means that doctors stimulated her ovaries to release *almost three years' worth of eggs at one time*). Of those eggs, fifteen were fertilized by a procedure called intracytoplasmic sperm injection (ICSI), where the technicians select individual sperm to inject directly into each egg. Since life begins at fertilization, that means that they became parents to fifteen children. After three days, however, they were told that only twelve of the embryos were viable, which indicates that there was already a loss of three children. They then were told that of the remaining embryos, five were "really good." Since the doctors were only going to insert two embryos, the couple said that they would freeze at least three, while the clinic would watch the development of the remaining embryos in vitro to see if they would freeze more. (In the end, a total of five were frozen.) By inserting only two, anyone concerned about the safety of the youngest humans among us must ask: *What will be the fate of the remaining ten children?* Freezing five of them is an attempt to preserve some of them (and the couple expressed wanting to pursue IVF again), but that process of freezing itself is not without consequence and risk to the tiny children, as we'll see below. Moreover, what of the other five children?

The couple was happy to report that the two embryos inserted into the wife's body successfully implanted, and she gave birth months later to fraternal twin girls. But their story is not just about creating two lives. It is also about those *thirteen other lives*, the rest of whom are either already dead or stuck in a freezer.

Humans were meant to develop on a specific timeline. Our species, for example, needs approximately nine months in the womb (whereas, by contrast, elephants need almost two years). When we freeze preborn humans, we are ceasing their ability to grow and develop along a normal trajectory. If we wait, for example, five or ten years before thawing and implanting them, we are denying them the right to grow up alongside the peers they would naturally grow up with. In other words, when a ten year frozen embryo (based on her conception date) is born, she should actually be growing up alongside preteens, not infants. Or take the case of an actual frozen embryo who was transferred and brought to term: that human was in a freezer for twenty-four years, meaning that when she was actually born, she should have been in a university, not a nursery.

Besides the injustice of denying a human her right to mature on a timeline that accords with her nature, freezing embryos risks a child's ability to survive. According to Dr. Sonya Kashyap, former medical director of Genesis Fertility Centre and a clinical assistant professor at the University of British Columbia, "80 to 90 per cent of embryos survive the thawing process." That means 10 to 20 percent of frozen embryos do not survive the thawing process. The Utah Fertility Center previously reported a greater success rate: "Approximately 95% of embryos typically will survive the freeze-thaw process." Setting aside the uncertainty introduced by words like "approximately" and "typically," this still means that as a best estimate for these fertility centers, 5 percent of embryos *will not* survive. This leads to a fundamental question: *Is it ethical to endanger the lives of some children in an effort to create other children?*

In the United Kingdom, Parliament reported that between 1991 and 2015, more than 2.3 million embryos were discarded for the 1.7 million embryos that were transferred. It's been estimated that the United States has one million human beings in freezers. Some of those may be retrieved for a transfer attempt, but others will be left frozen with annual payments covered by their parents, and still others will be abandoned entirely.

Some embryos are not selected for freezing at all because they are deemed genetically unfit, and thus they are killed. (They are exposed to environments they cannot survive in and discarded as medical waste.) Other embryos are experimented on until they die because their parents chose to "donate" them to research. In fact, embryonic stem cell research uses many of these leftover embryos.

And even when embryos are transferred to a woman's body, some styles of IVF involve transferring more embryos than would be safe to gestate, if all happened to implant.

One fertility clinic shared the testimony of a woman who went through three cycles of IVF in which she had six children transferred each time, for a total of eighteen offspring. In the end, however, she only birthed two of the eighteen, so it seems the other sixteen did not succeed in implanting. But what if all six children had implanted at one time? What if some or all of them became identical twins and doubled her pregnancy to twelve? (Identical twins form when one embryo splits into two, whereas fraternal twins form when two eggs are fertilized by two sperm.) A twin pregnancy is already a high-risk pregnancy. Having three, four, or more babies in utero is dangerous. Fertility clinics may try to avoid this by only implanting one or two embryos, but not always. Sometimes they transfer larger quantities because they expect the odds are low that all will implant and grow. But what if the unexpected actually happens?

If it does, it is common for the fertility industry to recommend a "selective reduction" abortion, where a doctor will kill several children in utero to increase the odds of one or two developing safely to term. A fertility clinic describes this as follows: "If multiple pregnancies occur, a multifetal selective reduction procedure can be considered. This procedure is performed at approximately ten weeks of pregnancy and involves injecting a salt solution into one or more of the gestational sacs." That salt solution is essentially a poison intended to kill the targeted children.

As the above demonstrates, IVF harms humans in multiple ways:

1. It puts the youngest among us, at their most vulnerable age, outside of the safety of their mother's body and in an environment of a petri dish or a freezer, which involves a significant risk of death. (Note: Some might object by saying that the womb is not always safe, as miscarriage is a possibility. The difference between miscarriage and loss of life through IVF is that miscarriage is something that happens through no fault of one's own. By contrast, IVF purposefully puts the preborn in an environment where they are not meant to be and may not survive as a result.)
2. It kills embryos that are deemed unfit.
3. It kills embryos by way of using them for scientific research.
4. It kills embryos or fetuses through selective reduction abortion.

Consider the language of the Human Fertilisation and Embryology Authority in the United Kingdom. Regarding unused or leftover embryos, it declares, "Some people prefer to dispose of their embryos. Embryos that are no longer needed are simply removed from the freezer and allowed to *perish* naturally in warmer temperatures or water." The dictionary defines perish as "to become destroyed or ruined: cease to exist." If we are making someone cease to exist, that means that they *did* exist before our actions led to their demise.

There is no denying that the procedure of IVF can harm preborn humans. But it can harm born humans too.

6

Harming Born Humans

The Center for Bioethics and Culture Network is a research and advocacy organization that has become an authority on the harms of the fertility industry. Their documentary *Breeders* features the story of a surrogate who allowed her eggs to be used for the conception of a child who would be raised by a homosexual couple. The parties agreed that she could stay in touch with the child. She shared a striking story of how, when that little girl was visiting at the age of five, she was very focused on looks. Being raised by two men, but having been told that the woman she visited was her genetic mother, she remarked on all the physical similarities between herself and the surrogate. She also observed that the children the surrogate had with her husband actually looked less like their mom (because in certain ways they were more like their dad). Her little five-year-old mind led her to say, "We have the same hair and we have the same eyes. Why did you give me away and keep them?"

We should not underestimate the emotional, psychological, spiritual, and physical tolls that IVF has on those conceived as a result of it. In fact, there is a growing online presence of those who have been called "donor-conceived" children who struggle deeply with their origins and roots.

Some, for example, will never know their genetic parent(s), which means they will lack significant medical history that could be of benefit to them. For example, my friend's husband's mother got cancer and tested positive for the dangerous BRCA2 gene. As a result of that, her son (my friend's husband) got tested, and his results also came back positive. That puts him at high risk of developing cancers (prostate, melanoma, pancreatic, and even breast) at a young age. He is in his early thirties, and this knowledge gives him an opportunity to make serious lifestyle and health changes to decrease the likelihood of the gene expressing itself. The genetics counselor he met with even asked for a full family history for two generations—how everyone died, etc.—to get a full picture of what he is most at risk for. But what if he had been donor-conceived and denied knowledge of his genetic parents? The results could be disastrous. Some might say that he could just be proactively investigated for disease. However, there are an endless number of diseases a given individual could have, and without insight into a strong connection to justify testing, it would not make sense to do investigation after investigation. Moreover, some donor-conceived children are not informed that the parents raising them are not their biological parents, so they may truly be misinformed about their genetic background.

Donor-conceived children have even expressed worry that they are at risk of falling in love with a genetic half-sibling without realizing it. That is not an irrational fear; one man wrote about that very discovery in his own life. He and his wife were both raised by lesbian mothers. The wife was very curious about her biological father, so she contacted the sperm bank where he contributed and found out her paternity. This was important to her because she wanted to know her genetic roots for the sake of the children they would have. The husband, however, did not have an interest in finding out about his father and initially chose not to inquire. But one day, as a present to his wife, he decided that he, too, would search out his genetic father. And when he did, he was horrified to discover that he and his wife had the same dad. As he wrote, "I can't help but think 'This is my sister' every time I look at her now."

Revelations like that are catastrophic. But they are not the only wounds. Alana Newman is donor-conceived and shares the story of how, when she was a young child, her mother informed her that the man raising her was not her biological father. Alana naturally became curious about the sperm donor her mom had used to create her, but her mom's response was dismissive: "He doesn't matter." An interview with Alana about her story points out the obvious next question that can go through a child's mind: "Do *I* matter?"

Consider what happened a short while after that conversation: Alana's mom divorced from her husband, and although the husband did not have biological paternity to Alana or her adopted sister from Korea, he only stayed in touch with Alana's adopted sibling. Imagine the impact that had on the mind of eight-year-old Alana. As the *Irish Times* reported in an interview with her, "Newman describes this as the man's 'symmetrical' relationship with his adopted daughter, who is equally related (or unrelated) to both parents. Newman, on the other hand, is 'more' her mother's child."

Alana has since created an online community in which people conceived through technology can share the impact it has on them. At AnonymousUs.org, there are moving posts from people who express anguish about not knowing their biological families. One person wrote the following about finding her biological father at the age of twenty-six:

> I wish I even knew how to describe how wonderful and awful it has been all at the same time. Absolutely no relatives that I found have wanted a relationship with me. My biological father wouldn't even provide me with medical history. My grandma agreed to meet me, but then ghosted me. And my siblings haven't really wanted to talk. But to see my bio father's face and to know little things about him has been exactly what I've been longing for for many years, but it has also been so heartbreaking to know I can't even have a conversation with him after all this. I've gone through many difficult things in my life, but nothing can prepare you for rejection from your father. . . . The grief that I experience is very real. It may not make sense to people who aren't in my position, but I never knew it was possible for these losses to be as devastating as they are.

Another technology-conceived person posted,

> I have an abusive single mother who bought me to fill her loneliness, with her (conditional) love being contingent on meeting her needs. I have a donor-father who openly admits he helped bring me into this world so he could profit off of my existence and play out his Genghis Khan-like fantasy.
>
> These aren't matters of interpretation. These are unfortunately just the facts about my conception. And I am stuck with them. For the rest of my life, I am stuck with them. My healing

> will have to be a full acceptance of these facts, rather than having the ability to redo my thinking. I can be grateful to be alive all I want. It does not take away that people bought and sold me for their self-serving desires.

That last sentiment is key. Some people may say that because they are happy to be alive, they hesitate to criticize the circumstances of their conception; they acknowledge that they would not exist unless those circumstances happened. However, as the testimony above shows, one should not have to validate sin. God, in his majesty, can draw great things from our sin, but he never gives his stamp of approval to the sin itself. My friend Ryan, who was conceived in rape, is very happy to be alive, but in no way would he ever claim the circumstances of his conception were good. Moreover, sinful circumstances surrounding one's beginning can do lasting damage to a person's sense of well-being.

Indeed, what the aforementioned examples show is a negative impact on many people created by reproductive technologies, even if not everyone with that experience admits it. To the extent that we care about our fellow humans, particularly vulnerable children, we must not overlook this.

Consider Katy Faust. She created an organization called Them Before Us (and wrote a book by the same name) to "advance social policies that encourage adults to actively respect the rights of children rather than expecting children to sacrifice their fundamental rights for the sake of adult desires." In writing to the New York government about the harms of surrogacy on children, she said, "Donor children struggle disproportionately with depression, delinquency, and substance abuse. Eighty percent of donor-conceived children desire to know the identity of their biological father." Katy and her organization have done extensive research on what helps children flourish—and what harms them. Through studies and stories, they show how children created by IVF face various challenges and harms, thereby giving a voice to those struggling to be heard.

7

The Nature of Parenthood

A few years ago, the twelve-year-old son of one of my friends got so sick he required hospitalization. The boy's mom and dad were almost continually at his bedside. On a few occasions when they were not, they left confident that he was in good hands and would be well cared for. Children's hospitals typically have charities that facilitate as much parent-child closeness as possible by providing accommodations so parents do not have to travel far to be near their hospitalized child (something this couple took advantage of). Moreover, while a nurse or doctor can provide medical expertise and consolation, nothing beats a mother's or father's love and presence.

Contrast that with how frozen embryos are treated: these youngest and most vulnerable humans among us are left in cold freezers at temperatures as low as –320 degrees Fahrenheit. They are left there by their parents, sometimes for days, months, years, or forever. In fact, one fertility doctor in Fort Myers, Florida, reported, "Twenty one percent of our embryos have been abandoned." NBC News reported, "A paper co-authored in the scientific journal *Nature Biotechnology* by Dr. Arthur Caplan, one of the nation's leading bioethicists and a professor at the New York University

Medical School, stated there are at least 90,000 frozen embryos considered abandoned in the US. Other studies indicate the number is much higher, possibly in the millions."

These children are denied—temporarily or permanently—the safety and security of being nestled beneath their mothers' hearts. Some might respond that if it was okay for my friend to temporarily leave her son in the safety of the hospital, could parents temporarily leave their embryos in the safety of IVF clinics, especially because the embryos are unaware of their separation from their parents? The answer is no, and to understand why, consider the following: Would parents leave their children alone in a hospital that considered either caring for that child or killing that child to be equal options? Would parents leave their children alone in a hospital that intentionally weeded out children it deemed unhealthy or less desirable? Clearly not. And yet, the very nature of your average IVF clinic is that it will kill some preborn children or, where legally permitted, do research on preborn children, all in an effort to create other preborn children.

Fertility clinics are typically involved with pre-implantation genetic diagnosis, described as follows by the Reproductive Partners Medical Group: "This technology allows doctors to select embryos free of a specific genetic problem in order to create healthy babies." When doctors do that, it means they do *not* select embryos that *have* a specific genetic problem, making destruction the fate for those other embryos.

To see how extreme this can get, consider a new company called Orchid. Promoting their screening services, they explain, "Orchid sequences over 99% of an embryo's DNA, while alternatives sequence less than 1%." They proudly reveal how they can screen embryos for conditions like autism, epilepsy, pediatric hereditary cancers, and hearing loss, to name a few. They offer that they can screen IVF-created embryos for more than 1,200 "single gene" conditions. They advertise, "Find the embryo at lowest risk for a disease that runs in your family," which implies that the embryos at highest risk for such a disease are to be avoided. Indeed, in its Frequently Asked Questions section, Orchid writes, "When you conceive at home, random chance determines your child's genetics. When you create embryos through IVF, you can potentially forecast your child's genetics, choosing the healthiest of several possible embryos."

This doesn't sound like "survival of the fittest," but rather "destruction of the most unfit." After all, if you're "choosing" the most healthy, then that means you're *not* choosing the unhealthy. So what becomes the fate of the latter? Will the embryos with a poor genetic profile always be destroyed? I suppose not necessarily. It is possible that parents would try for such embryos to be implanted. But is it likely? Orchid says, "Based on the embryos' genetic health, patients and their care team can select the embryo with the lowest genetic risk and the best chance of IVF success. The remaining embryos can be frozen for future use." It is, however, worth considering how likely such "future use" is: If someone is so worried about their child having a certain condition that they are willing to spend more than $12,000 getting a genetic profile of their embryos (on top of the expense of the IVF process itself), why would they consider "using" the lesser-desired embryos down the road? Creating a bunch of children, subjecting them to fitness testing, and then choosing the healthiest hardly bodes well for those whose genetic profile doesn't make the first cut.

Criticism of genetic testing should not be interpreted as opposition to modern medicine. We live in a broken world, and sickness and disability are signs of something gone wrong; as will be discussed in chapter 12, it is good to want to restore our bodies to the healthy state they were designed to have. The problem with genetic testing of embryos so as to choose the "healthiest" is that the guiding principle isn't about restoring a sick or disabled body to a healthy state; it isn't about identifying an illness so as to eliminate it. Instead, it is about identifying already-existing people who may have poorly functioning bodies so as to avoid them. Such genetic tests don't lead people to correct "bad" genetics but instead influence them to avoid or even destroy an unwell child while nurturing the healthy siblings. It is certainly not reflective of how parents ought to behave toward their children.

The IVF industry is not primarily guided by children's interests but instead by parents' desires. Consider an article by Slate called "The Parents Who Want Daughters—and Daughters Only." It reports on people pursuing IVF, some of whom have no known infertility challenges, so that they can choose the sex of their embryo. IVF clinics are calling this "family balancing," so that if a couple has a child of one sex, they can work to intentionally create the opposite. The Fertility Institutes, an organization that has existed for over three decades, promotes this as a service, offering to help clients "Select the Gender and Eye Color of Your Next Baby."

Take the example of Paris Hilton. In January 2023, she and her husband welcomed a baby boy they created via IVF and had gestated via a surrogate. Of their pursuit of such technology, Hilton said, "And we've done it seven times. I have all boys. I have twenty boys." What will become of those many embryonic boys? It is unknown, but clearly at the top of her list was having a girl, as less than a year later they welcomed the birth of a daughter, also via IVF and surrogacy. Sometimes the desire isn't to balance one's family but to *only* have children of one sex. One person the Slate article references is a thirty-one-year-old woman who is creating and freezing embryos with her fiancé. She said, "When I think about having a child that's a boy, it's almost a repulsion, like, *Oh my God, no*."

The IVF industry is one that manufactures and uses young humans to meet the wishes of older humans. And that mentality infects all that they do. Not only can many children of one sex be created in order to obtain children of the other sex, not only are some genetically unfit children destroyed, but genetically fit children may be intentionally selected for their usefulness. A fertility center writes, "The couple may have a child or other family member who needs compatible stem cells to save that family member's life. In this case, embryos that possess a desirable genetic trait, such as a tissue type that matches an ailing sibling or other family member, can result in a child to provide cord blood stem cells." With this motivation, no longer is the human person valued for his or her uniqueness and nature of being an image-bearer; instead, the person is valued, wanted, and selected for the usefulness they provide to others.

To see how IVF is not compatible with how parents ought to view their own offspring, consider the story of journalist Elissa Strauss and her husband. They, their dog, and two of their children live in California, while two of their other children live in New

York—as frozen embryos. The Strausses already got what they wanted: an IVF-conceived child brought to term. Given that they created multiple children to achieve that one child, the question became this: What to do with their remaining embryos? When writing about their options, Elissa commented, "Embryos are useful." And right there is the problem. Children should not be viewed based on usefulness. That is not the language of love. Parenthood ought to be about the good of the child, but IVF turns things upside down so it is about the perceived good of the parent—at the expense of the child (or multiple children).

Moreover, because IVF allows for control and perfection in a way that natural conception does not, IVF can feed these tendencies in a parent so that they become obsessions. The pursuit of control and perfection even become gods; they are put on the highest pedestal, above the child herself, so that IVF is not so much about receiving a unique child but is instead about making a perfect baby, at the perfect time, at any cost. The human relationship of parent to child is no longer about awe and reverence toward this or that very specific, unrepeatable, irreplaceable, priceless—and yet imperfect—individual, but instead about making and grasping at an individual who works with the mold one has created of what one wants.

For example, in the documentary *#BigFertility: It's All About the Money*, an American surrogate shares her story of agreeing to gestate twins for a couple from Spain. The couple wanted a boy and a girl, and paid $5,000 extra to ensure a female embryo would be transferred with a male embryo. But as it happened, the female embryo died and the male embryo split into identical twins. The

Spanish couple was horrified to learn their surrogate was pregnant with two boys instead of a boy and a girl. The reality is that the couple paid for a girl and they wanted a girl, and what they were going to get simply did not fit their "order." Sadly, that attitude is not reflective of how parents should view their offspring.

Returning to the story of Elissa and her husband, it perhaps should not be surprising, although it is profoundly tragic, that they opted to take their "useful" embryos and "donate" them to research—which means they will eventually be killed. While Elissa even acknowledged that at some future point they may want more children, she opted against keeping the preborn children they already created: "We concluded that should our tides shift and we decide we want to have another kid, we will try to have another kid. Even if that means going through IVF." Even if that means going through IVF—*again*. If embryos are useful, there is no need to let old ones linger. Just start fresh and use new ones.

With infertility, what can begin as an understandably profound and deep-seated ache for children can, particularly with IVF, become twisted and distorted. When a natural desire turns into an obsession, it very quickly causes one to lose sight of true love, of reverence for persons, of receiving and accepting the other, and of the self-sacrificing nature of parenthood.

Consider what one mother said who pursued IVF and had remaining embryos:

> In the bowels of Midtown Manhattan, a trio of embryos sit in a vat of liquid nitrogen. They're the genetic siblings of my sons, Jack and Charlie, the frozen fruits of an IVF cycle completed in 2016—and I have no clue what to do with them. . . .

> For those like me who are definitely done reproducing (two kids is plenty for us, thanks), there are three options: preserve, discard, or donate. . . .
>
> And so, like many others, we're keeping our embryos on ice—not just pausing their chance at life but freezing time on the need to decide.

The attitude she expresses as a parent is one that would not be tolerated if she were speaking about born children. As pointed out by Abort73.com, "The highest expression of love has long been defined as a willingness to lay down your life for another. The opposite of laying down your life for another is to lay down another's life for your own."

Some might interject and say the examples given are not reflective of all couples who pursue IVF. Some might say that the attitudes of the people above are indeed objectionable, but that other parents might not be so callous. Others might propose that they would not opt for a pre-implantation genetic diagnosis and instead accept a disabled child. They might add that they plan on returning as quickly as possible to rescue their frozen embryos and simply need the freezing services as a type of daycare until the woman's body is ready for another pregnancy. Still others might pursue IVF by only creating one or two embryos with no plans to ever subject their children to a freezer.

Does having better intentions than someone else, by itself, make an action moral? It is entirely possible for someone to commit a wrong action but have good motivations. (For example, it is a wrong action to steal someone's wallet even if you intend to donate the money to the poor.) There is, within the whole system of IVF, an overarching attitude that is not compatible with how parents ought to view and treat their children. Even if there seem to be exceptions to this industry norm, there are still problems to be addressed.

8

The Commodification of Humans

Several years ago, after I spoke to a thousand-person crowd, an audience member approached me and shared that she was conceived by IVF. She told me in no uncertain terms that while she loves her life, she does not agree with how she came to be. "My mom doesn't understand," she said to me. "She doesn't see how I can be against the very thing that made me exist." She added, "I've seen the paperwork. *We were all just numbers.*"

Take a friend of mine whose sister-in-law pursued IVF. She learned through the process that embryos are graded just like essays in school. My friend's sister-in-law said, "We only have a C embryo left; we used the A and B ones already, so we aren't very optimistic." As one fertility clinic writes about this categorization process on its website, "During the in vitro fertilization (IVF) process, embryos created in the lab are graded by the embryology team to determine which embryos have the best appearance under the microscope. Fertility clinics grade embryos with different nomenclature, but each grading system enables the team to distinguish between good, average, and poor quality embryos in order to choose the embryo for transfer which has the highest chance of becoming a baby."

One of the problems with IVF is that it treats human beings as commodities, as objects. Whether it is nameless numbers, letter grades, or phrases like "poor-quality embryo," a system is used to refer to preborn humans in a way we simply do not refer to born humans. Consider this language from Genesis Fertility Centre, which has since shut down: "We are now proud to be perfecting the use of elective single embryo transfer (eSET). . . . Using eSET we're able [to] select a single *perfect* embryo." What happens if a child is less than "perfect"? If such children aren't weeded out before transfer as a result of pre-implantation genetic testing, then they may be killed in the womb. The *Daily Mail* in the UK reported that some IVF-conceived children who were found to have Down syndrome, for example, were aborted.

In the documentary *Breeders*, several women who chose to be surrogates tell their stories. One of those women found out at a twenty-one-week ultrasound that the child she was carrying for a couple had a severe brain deformity. The biological parents' response was that of people who view life as a commodity: they wanted the surrogate to abort their child (which she refused to do). When we humans purchase or order items that are defective, our response is to return them, either expecting our money back or an undamaged replacement. But humans are not items to be returned or discarded. And so wanting an abortion in the face of a child with special needs conveys that the child is not viewed as a subject but instead is viewed as an object.

IVF manifests a type of commodification of humans in all kinds of ways. Consider this language from the Society for Assisted Reproductive Technology (SART): "You can donate your embryos to another woman with fertility problems." We donate clothes to a thrift store; we donate paintings to a museum; but how is it ethical to "donate" a fellow human we ought not to own? After all, if a slave owner decided to "donate" his slave to another plantation, wouldn't we be just as outraged as if he *sold* that slave? Wouldn't we acknowledge that either approach treats the slave—a human being—as though she is a possession owned by someone else?

Some might raise a question here about the adoption of born children. Isn't adoption like embryo donation? First, when placing a child for adoption, society does not use the language of "donation." Adoption agencies do not say, "You can donate your infant to other adults," because a donation is an object and infants are subjects. Moreover, when making a donation, the orientation is about *who is receiving the donation*. Adoption is very different: it is about *who is in need of caregivers*.

Further, it is worth pointing out that adoption, while a beautifully generous gesture, is actually not ideal. As one of my friends, an adoptive mom, said, "I think all adoption stories have an element of sadness in them because in order to have adoption at least one party has experienced loss." What is ideal, then, is that children be raised in a loving home by their biological parents. But we do not live in an ideal world. Having said that, a woman who chooses adoption is not intentionally getting pregnant with the express purpose of placing the resulting child for adoption. Instead, a woman who chooses adoption is not intending to get pregnant but does. Then, once the child exists, she discerns that an adoptive couple could provide for her child better than she could herself.

IVF is very different. No child yet exists at the beginning of the process. It is only because the parents want to optimize the chance of a successful pregnancy that they typically have more children created than they would ever want or be able to birth. Promoting embryo "donation" then becomes a helpful way for fertility clinics to rationalize what they do because it appears altruistic. A child created by IVF and then donated is treated as an insurance policy. She is intentionally made as a backup. Adoption is ordered to the needs of the child, whereas IVF is ordered to the wants of the parents.

As we can see, embryo "donation" is very different from adoption. But sometimes the former isn't chosen at all; if a couple opts against implanting some of their embryos in another woman's womb, then SART explains the other options: "You can donate your embryos for laboratory research to help improve pregnancy rates for infertile couples in the future."

Consider the experimentation on Jews and others during the Holocaust: some humans were subjected to research with the justification that the information obtained would be helpful *for others*. What is completely overlooked is that it is not helpful *for the people experimented on*. The point of this analogy is not to compare those who mistreat humans but to compare various victim groups who are mistreated. Don't we raise a collective outcry against such actions because they treat humans as objects? Why then would we embrace that same philosophy with human beings who happen to be younger than Holocaust victims?

Another aspect of the fertility industry that reveals commodification but is often overlooked is the use of pornography in producing sperm samples. The Michigan Reproductive Medicine clinic spoke openly about this on their blog:

> We have 2 collection rooms here at Michigan Reproductive Medicine (or as we like to refer to them: Honeymoon Suite 1

> and 2). Inside the collection room, we have all the essentials for collecting a semen specimen: a vinyl "love" seat, a magazine rack with a variety of classic adult magazines, a television and DVD player with several adult movie options, a sterile collection cup, and a clipboard with paperwork for you to complete when you are finished collecting your sample. We also have Wi-Fi available for those who prefer to use their own device.

This means that people who are being used for the sex industry (with or without their consent) are being used in the IVF industry for the creation of a baby that is not their own. This also means a child's very beginnings will be connected not with an act of love-making between husband and wife but with an act of self-pleasuring of a lone man with the aid of nameless bodies on a screen.

The commodification culture of IVF continues: it is also manifested in the exchange of huge sums of money between the various parties involved as well as the involvement of sperm and egg sellers/donors and surrogates. Consider this blog from the Phoenix Sperm Bank:

> With the COVID-19 pandemic still affecting so much of our lives, including making a living, you may be looking for opportunities to earn extra money in 2022. If so, becoming a sperm donor is a great way to consistently make up to $1,500 per month while making a positive difference in the lives of others.
>
> If you are selected as one of our donors, you'll get $100 cash for each approved donation you offer (and about 90% of all donations are approved), and you can donate up to three times per week. . . .

> You can earn even more when you refer your friends to us. You will get $200 if that person makes it into the donor program, and another $300 once his donations are released for distribution. And there is no limit on the number of referrals you can make, which further boosts your earning potential.

Here we see the language of "donate," which sounds philanthropic, and while some countries do not allow the sale of sperm, in other places the potential for earning huge sums of money makes it more accurate to refer to the men as "sperm sellers." Men who sell sperm get lower compensation per contribution, but they can more readily provide their samples at a high frequency.

Contrast that with women who sell their eggs or rent their bodies as surrogates: they do it less often, but the prospect for high earnings is massive. For example, in Beverly Hills, California, Bright Expectations is an egg "donation" agency. They advertise that their compensation schedule is slightly higher than average and that women can receive anywhere from $8,000 to $10,000 *per* donation cycle. They have phrases on their website like "Egg donation is fundamentally altruistic," calling it "an intrinsically selfless decision" that is "based on generosity." But let's be clear: when someone is earning enough money to buy a car, put a down payment on a house, help pay for college, or go on an exotic vacation (all examples the agency provides when appealing to women), the label "egg donor" is incredibly misleading; "egg seller" seems more accurate.

And as high as the income can be for egg selling, it is nothing compared to the whole-body renting that is involved with surrogacy. West Coast Surrogacy in California lists its surrogate compensation breakdown: Their out-of-state base pay is $65,000, and that doesn't include expenses or allowances. (Plus, if you're an "experienced" surrogate, your base is actually $20,000 higher.) Moreover, the website previously advertised that if the parents who commissioned the surrogate decide they actually want an abortion of the child they had created, the surrogate would be paid up to $10,000 to go ahead with destroying the child who was once desired.

Contracts are drawn up, lawyers are involved—there is no denying that baby-making in the IVF industry is big business. Moreover, the fertility industry, always looking to reduce costs, has sought out women overseas, where, for example, the poor in India will be hired to sell eggs and/or gestate a foreigner's child at a much-reduced rate from the West. Online searches and documentaries will introduce you to how dark this commodification of humans—both born and preborn—can get.

While some may shine a spotlight on the compensation people get in order to focus on the positive, these interventions are not without risk. Egg donors/sellers could develop ovarian hyperstimulation syndrome. There is also a concern that the hormone exposure from stimulating an egg seller's ovaries could increase a woman's risk of developing cancer.

Consider the story of Maggie Eastman. Over a ten-year period, beginning when she was in college, she sold her eggs ten times. On just one of those occasions, she produced twenty eggs—almost two years' worth. Then, when Maggie was only thirty-two years old, she was diagnosed with stage 4 invasive ductal carcinoma—a breast cancer that had spread to other parts of her body. She had no family history of cancer, and at her age, it was incredibly rare to develop it—except when you factor in the hormones she was exposed to from harvesting her eggs. As Maggie bluntly put it, "I feel like I was prostituted and kept in the dark about the possible toll on my health." But that wasn't all: a hysterectomy was required as part of her cancer treatment, which means that she will never bear her own children even though her eggs may have been used to make untold numbers of humans.

Surrogacy is not without risk either. A 2018 journal article from the Brazilian Society of Assisted Reproduction reported that "the meta-analysis revealed a statistically significant association between egg donation [pregnancies] and onset of preeclampsia. . . . Oocyte donation is associated with increased risk of preeclampsia in singleton pregnancies. Therefore, it is crucial to properly record and assess this finding when egg donation is the chosen assisted reproductive technology to attain pregnancy."

Jennifer Lahl, president of the Center for Bioethics and Culture (CBC) Network, described the risks of surrogacy this way: "The surrogate mother . . . think of her as an organ donor. She's pregnant with a foreign embryo. Our female bodies were never designed to carry other peoples' babies. So in surrogacy, you'll see a surrogate mother is going to be at higher risk of preeclampsia, maternal hypertension, [and] gestational diabetes."

Preeclampsia was the experience of a surrogate named Kelly Martinez, whose story is shared in the CBC's documentary *#BigFertility: It's All About the Money*. Not only did the condition endanger her life, but because of how that surrogacy pregnancy went, doctors have advised her that she should not have any more children.

Admittedly, these negative experiences aren't always the stories of people who get involved with the big business of IVF; others have only positive stories to tell. But here is the point: if humans are treated as commodities, then humans will be like products delivered to a store—sometimes they are delivered in pristine condition and are readily purchased from the shelves, but other times objects get damaged. Some might say that this is the cost of doing business. And if something truly is a business, then that is a fair response. We are left, then, with a haunting question: Should the creative capacity of human beings—both the personal life-giving potential in our gametes as well as the offspring we are parents of—ever be treated like a business?

PART 3
The Blueprint

9

Be Fruitful and Multiply

When God created Adam and Eve, he gave them a clear command: "Be fruitful and multiply, and fill the earth and subdue it" (Gen. 1:28). This creative power is preceded by God's blessing upon them. It is a great good. When God began again with Noah and his family, God gave them the same command—"Be fruitful and multiply, and fill the earth" (Gen. 9:1)—and it, too, was enveloped in a blessing.

Throughout the Scriptures, we see fertility as a great blessing: "Sons are indeed a heritage from the LORD, the fruit of the womb a reward. Like arrows in the hand of a warrior are the sons of one's youth. Happy is the man who has his quiver full of them" (Ps. 127:3–5).

Correspondingly, in the Bible, we see infertility as a profound suffering. For example, Hannah's womb is described as being "closed" (1 Sam. 1:5), and this was a cause of great inner turmoil. The Scriptures say, "She was deeply distressed and prayed to the LORD, and wept bitterly. She made this vow: 'O LORD of hosts, if only you will look on the misery of your servant, and remember me, and not forget your servant, but will give to your servant a male child, then

I will set him before you as a nazirite until the day of his death. He shall drink neither wine nor intoxicants, and no razor shall touch his head" (1 Sam. 1:10–11).

In light of this, it seems that creating children with the help of IVF would be living up to the command to "be fruitful and multiply," that it would be a solution to barrenness and a celebration of fruitfulness. Although on the surface that seems to be the case, if we dig a little deeper, we see that one should not be so quick to draw that conclusion.

Let's unpack this claim by considering the nature of sex. A sex drive is inherent to being an adult human. It is a sign that our bodies have reached maturity and an indicator that they are working correctly (which is why people may go to their doctors to address the problem of low libido). Identifying the nature of something is necessary, but not sufficient, in understanding how it should be used. Just because we have a sex drive does not mean we should act on it anytime, anywhere, with anyone. We need to also look at the nature of our sexuality through the lens of a moral code; in this case, we will look at it through a Christian worldview.

By way of analogy, when considering the nature of the eye, it is reasonable to conclude that it is designed to see. Therefore, if someone is blind, we can conclude the eye is not functioning as it should. But just because blindness is a pathology, does that mean that, if we have sight, we should see every single thing? It does not. For example, if we used our sight to peek through someone's curtains to watch their private activity, our eye is doing the "right" thing (according to its nature) by seeing, but this good is being misused to do something evil. In other words, we take the good thing of sight and apply it (according to a moral code) to the wrong thing—in this case, violating someone's privacy.

Likewise, when it comes to our bodies and sex, we need to look at nature *and* morality. So we have a sex drive, but how ought we to use it? From a Christian perspective, the only relationship in which sex is permitted is the permanent relationship of marriage. Looking at the nature of sex can help us understand why this is the case. When a couple engages in sexual relations, their bodies release bonding hormones that "attach" them to their partner in a way that they aren't bonded to others. Moreover, sex has the inherent power to create offspring. These two realities make sex inappropriate for nonexclusive, non-lifelong relationships because it is not healthy for individuals to bond so intimately only to have those bonds broken. The stronger a bond (and sex creates a strong bond), the stronger the pain when that bond is severed. Furthermore, in an ideal world, children should be raised in a loving home by both their mother and father, and that is less likely when the parents have not pledged a permanent union, thus creating instability for any offspring. And so, for the good of both the couple and any children they might produce, sex should only happen in marriage.

Since sex is how God created humans to reproduce, that means, by God's design, that the only way that children ought to come to be is through the one relationship where sex is allowed—marriage—and that children should only come about from the union of a husband's and wife's seeds (gametes). Ethicist and Catholic priest Fr. Tadeusz Pacholczyk has remarked,

> Our sex cells, or gametes, are special cells. They uniquely identify us. They are an intimate expression of our own bodily identity,

> and mark our human fruitfulness. Each of us, in fact, has been given a capacity, a radical capacity, for total self-donation to a unique member of the opposite sex in marriage. Our gametes, and their exclusive availability to our spouse through marital acts, manifest this beautiful and life-engendering possibility of giving ourselves away to the one person whom we singularly love.

Further to his point, sperm and eggs are different from, for example, skin cells. The latter is something that tells the story of us, but the former, when combined with the corresponding gamete from our beloved, is something that will tell the story of our shared offspring. Rev. Pacholczyk continues, "Hence, donating to sperm or egg banks violates something fundamental at the core of our own humanity. It dissociates us from the deeper meaning of our own bodies and gravely damages the inner order of the marital union."

In other words, we shouldn't give away our gametes the way we may give away our blood. Our gametes are meant to be united only with the gametes of the one person we have united with in the covenant of marriage. Thus, we can come to the conclusion that for a married couple to use a third party's sperm or egg to create offspring would be unethical, because that sort of gamete union in the lab would be—morally speaking—impossible to achieve in the marriage bed. The same is true with surrogacy: the presence of a preborn child in a woman's body is designed to come to be through sexual intimacy exclusive to spouses (more on that in the subsequent chapters). An act of sex between husband and wife would only bring about an embryo in the biological mother's body, not a surrogate's, so a third party shouldn't be enlisted to do what, yet again, the marriage bed would not morally allow for.

The command to be fruitful and multiply doesn't give us license to fulfill it in just any way; for example, we may not justify adultery on the grounds of fulfilling that directive. We are only supposed to be fruitful and multiply with our spouse. So that would immediately exclude sperm or egg sellers/donors as well as surrogates. This might lead someone to ask, "So is IVF acceptable with very narrow parameters that would include only the husband's and wife's gametes?"

10

Narrowing the Parameters

Someone might read what I have said so far and acknowledge the following:

- Embryos should never be created with gametes outside those of the married male's and female's gametes.
- Embryos should never be frozen.
- Embryos should never be killed.
- Embryos should not be valued based on a eugenics mentality, which means they should not be subjected to genetic testing where the unfit are weeded out.
- Embryos should not be created to be handed over to surrogates.
- An unsafe quantity of embryos should never be placed in the mother's body.

But such an individual might suggest that while IVF is generally problematic, under the following very narrow parameters it could be acceptable:

- Only one or two embryos are created from the gametes of the married male and female.

- The embryos are not tested for genetic "fitness" but embraced regardless of their health.
- The embryos are transferred to the body of their biological mother without being subjected to a freezer.

While such a perspective is certainly an improvement from how our culture practices IVF, it still has flaws. By way of analogy, if you're shooting arrows at a target, you might get closer to the bull's-eye on one try than on others, but if none hit the center, the arrows are still "off."

To understand why even these narrow parameters are problematic, let's begin by returning to an analogy in chapter 4 about gifts: the scenario of giving a store's toy to a child when you have not bought it and it is not your gift to give. What if we changed the scenario a bit? What if the store owner, who was friends with you, observed the same situation and said, "Look, I'm really busy right now, but I want to help that poor kid. Take this toy and give it to him when he walks out. I'll write it off in the books later." In that case, you aren't the gift giver; you are the gift deliverer. Couldn't those providing IVF view themselves as "delivering" God's gift of life to couples by using their rational minds and modern technology?

To answer that, we have to ask another question: Does it fit with God's designs about sexual intimacy to enlist a third party, outside of a married couple, when it comes to the very moment of creating new life? Recall from the previous chapter that what sets marriage apart from all other relationships is leaving and cleaving: "A man leaves his father and his mother and clings to his wife, and they become one flesh" (Gen. 2:24); it is the inclusion of sexual intimacy that bonds and (sometimes) bears babies. Certainly, in addition to having a sexual relationship, married couples also live under the same roof, share meals and finances, and talk about their hopes and fears, but nonmarital relationships can include those elements too. After all, siblings, cousins, and friends sometimes live under the same roof, share meals and finances, and talk about hopes and fears. But marriage, unlike these other relationships, is ordered toward sexual intimacy. Moreover, while a married couple may invite others into their home to share in meals and friendship, it would not be proper for a married couple to invite others into their home to share in their sexual activity, because that is supposed to be a private and intimate expression between the couple who have committed to being together "until death do us part." If it weren't for very recent technology, then sexual intimacy would be the only way for humans to generate offspring; one could say that generating children is inherent to a couple's sexual activity. By pursuing IVF, a couple is taking the life-creating element of their private, exclusive, one-flesh union and inviting in a third party. Granted, they are not doing that in the moment of sex itself, but they are nonetheless taking that element inherently attached to the climax of sex and contracting it out to individuals external to their union.

To be fair, a couple may find that there are times when they need to seek outside support to help their sexual activity achieve its ends, whether that is getting counseling if they are having trouble with emotional bonding or seeking medical help if their bodies aren't working properly (e.g., the husband needs pharmaceuticals to achieve an erection or the wife needs pharmaceuticals to ovulate). There is a vitally important distinction to be made here: in these situations, the couple is enlisting a third party *outside of the moments of bonding and life creation* to correct something that is wrong so that *when the couple is privately and exclusively in those moments*, they can more likely achieve babies with their bonding. This approach works with God's designs and ensures that the body and mind are in optimal condition to express and achieve what God has beautifully created for the husband and wife. Contrast that with IVF, where the couple is enlisting a third party in *the very moment of life creation* that is designed by God to occur in the sexual act, an act that is reserved only for the spouses.

Another way to look at it is this: When a couple studies how their bodies work and uses that knowledge to be sexually intimate at a time that is optimal for conception (e.g., they track precisely when the wife is ovulating), are they actually making a baby? They might use the phrase "let's make a baby," but at a technical level, even ideally timed sex doesn't make a baby. Instead, it creates an environment that is conducive to life *being created* while placing the couple in a type of receptive position.

Here is what I mean: If a woman shows signs of ovulation on Tuesday but her egg is not released until Thursday, and she and her husband have sex each day from Monday to Friday, which of those five acts of sex will contain the winning sperm? We do not know (because sperm can live for several days in a woman's body in the right conditions, such as with fertile-type cervical mucus). If the couple has sex at 8 a.m. on Thursday, does that mean they would have conceived in that very act? Not if the egg hasn't released yet, which means the wife might conceive that afternoon while driving to the hairdresser when a sperm, still alive in her body, successfully swims to the then-released egg.

This helps us see there is something about God's designs for a couple's ability to "be fruitful and multiply" that is both hands-on *and* hands-off. Yes, the couple is proactive by engaging in the marital act, but then they are receptive by waiting and seeing if life comes to be. And if it does, which sperm? Which egg? Which day? Which time? That is out of their hands. They aren't forcing someone into existence. They are receiving someone whom God brings into existence.

IVF, in contrast, is making someone; it is manufacturing a human person. No longer are the parents receiving new life as a fruit of their sexual intimacy; instead, a new human is beginning at the hands of a stranger. A scientist is bringing the sperm and egg together (sometimes, even, selecting one sperm to inject directly into an egg). IVF does not actually mimic what happens naturally; it changes it. The husband, instead of giving his seed to the one person he's meant to share it with—his wife—is handing it off to a stranger. The wife, instead of waiting in great expectation about whether her husband's seed will fertilize the egg in her body, has her eggs removed by a fertility clinic and waits for a report from them. The human child, in her most vulnerable and fragile state, begins life in a lab instead of beneath her mother's heart. This isn't to deny the deep ache of couples who desperately want a baby and feel that this is their only chance for that. They might not even be viewing IVF from this manufacturing perspective at all. It is instead to point out that good desires and even a lack of bad intentions do not automatically make for an ethical act.

God made sex necessary for new human life; IVF makes sex unnecessary. Sex receives humans that God creates; IVF manufactures humans. Sex unites; IVF separates.

Let's expand on this last point. In the first creation story, God says, "Let us make humankind in our image, according to our likeness" (Gen. 1:26). Who is "our"? If we believe in one God, then how can he be plural? The answer is that God is a communion of persons; he is a Trinity—the Father, the Son, and the Holy Spirit. That means that because of our nature as the image of God, we are made for a communion of persons. And we see that very specifically through sexual intimacy: of all our bodily systems (e.g., circulatory, respiratory), the one that is incomplete is the reproductive system. That system has only half of what it needs to be fully functioning; it requires another body.

In the second creation story, God says, "It is not good that the man should be alone; I will make him a helper as his partner" (Gen. 2:18). Of the various animals God then created, none were a match, until "the rib that the LORD God had taken from the man he made into a woman and brought her to the man. Then the man said, 'This at last is bone of my bones and flesh of my flesh'" (Gen. 2:22–23). And then we are told, "Therefore a man leaves his father and his mother and clings to his wife, and they become one flesh" (Gen. 2:24).

Sex is a communion of persons. It is no accident that image-bearers are given the blessing of creating more image-bearers through a process of what they image: a communion of persons. It is no accident that, in the natural order, a newly conceived human needs the body of her mother to mature, thereby also necessitating a communion of persons. Not all animals are designed to have life begin and be initially nourished in their mothers' bodies, but placental mammals are designed that way. Our very start involves never being alone; it involves a profound and intimate reflection of the Trinity of the Father, Son, and Holy Spirit through the father, mother, and child. IVF, in contrast, can be executed with the total separation of each person: the man typically masturbates to provide a sperm sample; the woman's eggs are retrieved in a medical clinic; the child begins her life in a glass dish. At a technical level, *none have to be together* for the creation to occur.

There is another point to consider. With sex between a husband and wife, there is absolutely no risk of any child being created except for the genetic offspring of that couple. Even with the best practices of an IVF clinic, however, there is always a risk of human error that the sperm of one patient is used to fertilize the wrong woman's egg (or vice versa), thereby creating someone who would never, morally speaking, be able to come into existence through the marital act.

This isn't a hypothetical. A couple from New Jersey sued the fertility clinic they used because when their daughter was two years old, she started showing signs of Asian features, which bewildered her Caucasian parents. They pursued DNA testing and discovered that the assumed biological father was actually not her dad. This is not an isolated incident. Two couples in the United States sued their fertility clinic because the genetic offspring of couple A was mistakenly implanted in the woman from couple B. An internet search reveals more tragic stories like these from around the world.

Recall the points in chapter 8 about the commodification of humans. Because humans are subjects and not objects, we should be created differently than objects. Objects are manufactured, a process that involves putting parts together using various peoples' skill, talent, and time. That is what IVF does. But subjects should not come to be in the same way because we are so radically different. As mentioned previously, those created by science have dignity just like those created by sex; in fact, it's precisely this dignity that makes manufacturing humans through IVF so wrong. Treating the subject as an object is an offense to that individual. It does not bestow the honor and respect due to persons. We humans have been granted an incredible power to partner with God in the creation of other human beings. When we are given the blessing and command to be fruitful and multiply, we are invited to participate in God's work of creating an ensouled body made in the image of the divine. This is profoundly sacred. It is a privilege that should cause us to bow our heads in reverence and awe at the mystery we are welcomed into. (For those yearning for this but struggling with infertility, there is hope, as outlined in chapter 12.) The key is that we must take great care to respect precisely how God designed this to happen—at his direction, as a fruit of the physical expression of marital love. It is not something to be redesigned by human hands and contracted out to scientists for manufacture.

11

Sacred Mystery

In 2002, I was twenty-two years old and beginning my pro-life speaking career. I presented at an international conference and, in the days following, participated in a formal abortion debate against a university professor. In both audiences, there was a man who introduced himself to me and signed up for my ministry newsletters. He had a long (and epic!) beard and wore a black robe called a cassock. On his head was a round black hat. Around his neck was a large metal Byzantine crucifix. I was to discover he was a Ukrainian Greek Catholic monk and priest. Over the years, Hieromonk Teodosy Kraychuk wrote me very encouraging letters to support my work and introduced me to friends of his, Fr. Roman and Irene Galadza, a Ukrainian Catholic priest and his wife. Getting to know them acquainted me with the Eastern Rite liturgy. At their Ukrainian Greek Catholic parish in Ontario, Canada, my heart and soul were opened to the otherworldly beauty and sacredness of the ancient liturgies of early Church Fathers St. Basil the Great (who died in 379) and St. John Chrysostom (who died in 407).

Their church, St. Elias the Prophet, was all wood and had onion domes. People of all faiths and backgrounds regularly drove up to take in the magnificent architecture with awe and wonder. When visitors would walk in, they would be hushed by the sense of the sacred. The smell of beeswax candles (the only form of lighting for the whole church, excepting oil lamps or sunbeams shining through windows) was sweet to the senses. The floor-to-dome artwork capturing biblical scenes had taken ten years for an artist from Ukraine to complete and was breathtaking to behold. Just as the temple in Jerusalem had a separate, veiled space called the Holy of Holies that was only to be entered by high priests, so too was there a sanctuary behind the icon screen that was shrouded from the view and presence of the general public.

Then there were the liturgies themselves—an entirely sensual experience: the sounds of bells and the chorus of voices raised in harmony (there was no choir, but everyone enthusiastically followed a cantor in song); the words and chants of the ancient liturgy; and the vestments of the priest, deacons, and others serving, which made me imagine the Jewish priests in a Hebrew temple. There were also the smells of incense and the taste of Communion. In every way, these realities drew the human experience to heights that went beyond this world. It was nothing like everyday life. It was mystical, even supernatural.

When the community slowly sang, "Let us who mystically represent the Cherubim, and sing the Thrice-holy Hymn to the life-giving Trinity, now lay aside all cares of life, that we may receive the King of all, escorted invisibly by ranks of angels. Alleluia, alleluia, alleluia," it felt as though a choir of angels had descended into this sacred space with Jesus, the Lamb of God himself, while lifting our hearts up to paradise. My mind was blown. I had experienced heaven on earth.

As I reflect on my experiences of mystery, awe, and reverence in both the building and liturgy of that Eastern tradition, I think about how so many of our churches and liturgies today lack the layers, the history, the sacred, the mystical, and the otherworldly experience that was present there. And I am led to this question: *Is it possible that, as we have lost the sense of the sacred in the temples of our church buildings and worship, we have correspondingly lost the sense of the sacred in the temples of our bodies?* Let's reflect on the temple by looking at the second chapter of John:

> The Passover of the Jews was near, and Jesus went up to Jerusalem. In the temple he found people selling cattle, sheep, and doves, and the money changers seated at their tables. Making a whip of cords, he drove all of them out of the temple, both the sheep and the cattle. He also poured out the coins of the money changers and overturned their tables. He told those who were selling the doves, "Take these things out of here! Stop making my Father's house a marketplace!" His disciples remembered that it was written, "Zeal for your house will consume me." (John 2:13–17)

Why was Jesus so outraged? Because he observed a misuse of the temple of God. The temple was to be a place of worship, prayer, sacrifice, and praise. *The temple was not to be used for purposes outside of its design.* The passage continues,

> The Jews then said to him, "What sign can you show us for doing this?" Jesus answered them, "Destroy this temple, and in three days I will raise it up." The Jews then said, "This temple has been

> under construction for forty-six years, and will you raise it up in three days?" But he was speaking of the temple of his body. (John 2:18–21)

Jesus' body was the new Temple. It was the dwelling place of God. And in Paul's First Letter to the Corinthians, we are reminded that we are temples too: "Do you not know that your body is a temple of the Holy Spirit within you, which you have from God, and that you are not your own? For you were bought with a price; therefore glorify God in your body" (1 Cor. 6:19–20). Since our bodies are temples, we are to use them as God designed—not as man desires.

We are meant to have great reverence when handling and interacting with the human body. That is why we have a duty to bury the dead and have laws against mistreating corpses. If that is our responsibility to a body that has no life, then how much more of a responsibility do we have for the body that is very much alive? No matter how careful a scientist may be, creating human life outside the mother's body puts the youngest of our kind in a dangerous place where they could be—and many times are—harmed. Moreover, it removes the element of mystery and sacredness that lies within the sexual act and its capacity to bear the fruit of another human being to whom God gives a soul. As my friend Kenneth said (whose story is told in chapters 1 and 12), "The fallopian tube where conception can happen is the God zone, and we shouldn't go there. We need to leave that space for God's grace to happen." IVF, however, makes the beginning of life a laboratory activity; as Jesus cried out, "Stop making my Father's house a marketplace!" (John 2:16).

Some might point out that sex is not necessary to create humans because three people were made without sex: Adam, Eve, and Jesus. Just because God can make humans without sex, it does not logically follow that this gives humans license to make other humans without sex (and specifically by science). Adam and Eve were the beginning of the human race, made directly and solely by God without human involvement. Since God doesn't have sex, it makes sense for him to create man as he did (and practically, since no humans existed prior to Adam and Eve, there were no humans to have sex to conceive them). In the case of Jesus being conceived without sex, by Mary being a virgin, there was no denying the divine origin of the Incarnation—that God, and no human male, was the Father. But notice that when Jesus did enter into the human experience, he still did so enveloped within the body of his mother. There still was a communion of persons. He was beneath her heart. There was mystery, receptivity, and a sense of the sacred.

The points fleshed out in the last two chapters can be summarized in the following chart:

Life from IVF	Life from making love
Man masturbates. Man is alone. *Man withholds seed from his wife's body.*	Man and woman cleave to one another, becoming one flesh. The couple is together. *Husband deposits seed into wife's body.* There is giving and receiving, a true communion of persons.
Woman's eggs are *retrieved* by a third party.	Woman's egg is hidden in the environment of her body and *receives* her husband's seed. No other human party is involved.
Embryo *begins life apart from her parents* in a glass dish in the presence of a stranger. The image-bearer's beginning is observed and not enveloped. *A stranger is witnessing the sacred, which should be shrouded, not exposed.* The embryo is in a dangerous and vulnerable position being outside of the environment created for her.	Embryo *begins life beneath her mother's heart.* The embryo is never alone. The image-bearer's beginning is not observed and is enveloped. The mystery of another human soul starting occurs away from human sight and yet at the same time within a maternal embrace. *The sacred is not seen, maintaining the mysteriousness of life's beginning.*

Life from IVF	Life from making love
Embryo is made as a direct result of a stranger putting the parents' parts together. Scientists might even select the sperm, thereby influencing which individual comes into being. *There is a manufacturing element*. Creature becomes creator.	*Embryo is "begotten, not made"*: The couple responds to conditions favorable to life beginning, but they do not "make" it happen; they do not force the union of sperm and egg. If sperm meets egg, which sperm meets egg these are beyond their control. Sperm-egg fusion occurs as a fruit of their act. Creature aids Creator.
Baby's creation is separate from the act of parental bonding. While the couple may love each other deeply, a new human life does not come into being through a physical manifestation of that love. *Science unleashes life.*	Baby comes into being through an act of parental bonding. The very act of the couple is a physical representation of their marital love for each other, and it is that which results in a new human life. *Love unleashes life.*

12

Shalom

On August 1, 2020, I got married—three weeks after my fortieth birthday. Getting married that late in life, I wondered how easy it would be to achieve a pregnancy that my husband and I keenly hoped to have.

Only two cycles into our marriage, my husband and I were overjoyed to conceive a little one in my womb. But that joy would quickly be replaced with sorrow as we lost our child, Laetificat ("LaeLae") Judah, to miscarriage midway through the first trimester.

We got pregnant again. And it was then when a friend said to me, "Have you had your progesterone tested? Some women are low in that, and if that is the case, it can lead to miscarriage." I thanked my friend but dismissed her comment as not being relevant to me. I had tracked my cycle for years and seemed to have a textbook body. Plus, our doctor had thought the miscarriage was because our baby was very disabled and stopped growing rather than something hormonally wrong with me.

Life went on until another friend also brought up progesterone testing. I similarly dismissed her suggestion with my explanation above. But then another friend mentioned it, and another—to the point that about five friends (all unrelated) raised the issue with me. I started to wonder if maybe I shouldn't be so flippant. I started to wonder if the constant questioning was a sign meant to help me. So I called my doctor and had my progesterone checked. My levels were good, and I breathed a sigh of relief.

But I am a thorough person. Out of an abundance of caution, I asked my physician to test my progesterone one more time the following week, to make sure the level was climbing at the expected rate. Seven days later, my husband and I were horrified to discover that not only had my progesterone *not* gone up, it had gone down. Fearing another miscarriage, we immediately sought out a physician who is a specialist in natural fertility awareness and in the monitoring of progesterone to achieve and maintain a pregnancy. He is part of a network of doctors trained in what is called NaProTechnology. Developed by Dr. Thomas Hilgers, a clinical professor in the Department of Obstetrics and Gynecology at Creighton University School of Medicine in Omaha, Nebraska, "Natural Procreative Technology is a women's health science that monitors and maintains a woman's reproductive and gynecological health. It provides medical and surgical treatments that cooperate completely with the reproductive system. . . . Unlike common suppressive or destructive approaches, NaProTechnology works cooperatively with the procreative and gynecologic systems. When these systems function abnormally, NaProTechnology identifies the problems and cooperates with the menstrual and fertility cycles that correct the condition, maintain the human ecology, and sustain the procreative potential."

My NaPro-trained physician prescribed progesterone capsules and continued to supervise my levels. They increased, but then they decreased, so he adjusted my dosage accordingly, regularly having my blood tested for progesterone, which I needed to take until I was twenty-three weeks pregnant.

Just because IVF has been ruled out, morally, as a response to infertility, it does not follow that there is nothing to be done. A couple can investigate whether there are conditions of either the man or woman that can be corrected at their root. After all, if there is an ailment or pathology, it is good to treat it so as to restore the body to the healthy state God designed it to have. Opposing IVF is about opposing the manufacturing of image-bearers, but it is not about opposing medical advancement and intervention. Another way to put it is this: while using science and technology to produce a whole *person* is rejected, using science and technology to restore a body *part* to its proper function is entirely reasonable and good. In the Scriptures, we see Jesus healing peoples' ailments: the man blind from birth to whom Jesus gave sight (John 9:1–12), the centurion's servant lying paralyzed whom Jesus healed (Matt. 8:5–13), and Peter's mother-in-law from whom Jesus removed a fever (Matt. 8:14–15), to name a few. In Matthew 9:35, we are told that "Jesus went about all the cities and villages . . . curing every disease and every sickness." What we see is Jesus restoring the body to its healthy function. In contrast, IVF seeks to override, to change God's designs—and that is where the problem lies. But medical interventions, like administering progesterone, that restore the body to its right-ordered design are good.

This idea of restoration ties into the concept of *shalom*. Dr. Anne Bradley describes it well when she writes, "In the Old Testament, the concept of flourishing is best described by the Hebrew word *shalom*. Biblical scholars tell us that shalom signifies a number of things, including salvation, wholeness, integrity, soundness, community, connectedness, righteousness, justice, and well-being. Shalom denotes a right relationship with God, with others, and with God's good creation. It is the way God intended things to be when he created the universe. In most of our English Bibles, we translate shalom as peace, but it means much more than just an absence of conflict."

Because we are living in a broken world that involves sickness and disease, our bodies and relationships don't always match up to the ideal. But this gives us an opportunity to reweave *shalom*, to work toward reestablishing things as they should be. It involves right order and right relationship with God, with our neighbor, and in our designs. Pursuing corrective interventions that address infertility at its root leads to human flourishing and restores the body to God's designs of fertility; all the while, it maintains the sacredness of sexual intimacy between spouses as God intended it to be.

When Dr. Jonathan T. Pennington writes about the concept of *shalom*, he points out that the word functions in three main ways in the Old Testament:

1. In standardized greetings and partings, even as today we say "Peace" or "Peace to you" (about 10% of the uses).
2. To refer to a state or relationship that is peaceful, that is, free from conflict or tension (about 25% of the uses).
3. To refer to completeness, maturity, and especially overall well-being economically, relationally, healthwise (about 65% of the uses).

Note that it is this third usage that is the most common. The spirit of *shalom* should inspire us to work toward overall health and wellness, to maintain relationships as God designed.

In light of this, there are alternatives to IVF that demonstrate *shalom*. For example, if a woman is not releasing eggs, it can be ethical to prescribe her a pharmaceutical to prompt her body to ovulate. Doing so would restore her body to the normal, healthy function it is supposed to have. Doing so would *aid* the sexual act in achieving a pregnancy but *not replace* the sexual act like IVF does. If a lack of ovulation is identified as the problem, it is important to bear in mind that where medicine is administered to help a woman ovulate, it should only be given in a dose that would cause her body to release no more than one or two eggs. Hyperstimulating her ovaries so that an unnatural number of eggs are released could result in all the eggs being fertilized from an act of sex.

This was something my friends Mariam and Kenneth (mentioned in chapter 1) learned the hard way. They have never conceived in the entirety of their marriage, but they certainly tried. One of the fertility approaches they pursued was superovulation, whereby Mariam gave herself injections in her abdomen to prompt her ovaries to release eggs. A doctor told them that on ultrasound, it showed she had five eggs that would be available, so they could go home and have sexual relations. Mariam asked, "What if I get pregnant with five?" and the doctor replied, "Not to worry; we will just reduce you." Sadly, as mentioned in chapter 5, some medical professionals consider aborting some preborn children to be acceptable when a large number have successfully implanted. Not wanting to risk Mariam's life or health, or the life or health of their children should she have actually conceived more than one, they abstained from sex that cycle. But that meant that a whole round of fertility treatment went down the drain because of a physician who mismanaged her treatment.

My friend Lea got married at thirty-nine. As much as she and her husband hoped to conceive, she had lower expectations due to her age. Within six months they got pregnant but sadly miscarried their child at the end of the first trimester. That opened Lea's eyes to the idea that she wasn't too old to get pregnant. But she would face another miscarriage and a couple of years of no pregnancies before finally giving birth to a daughter a month shy of her forty-third birthday.

It was discovered through a blood test that Lea has antiphospholipid syndrome (APS), which is a clotting condition that, without shots to thin a woman's blood and make it less likely to clot, could otherwise cause a miscarriage. It explained her previous two miscarriages, and she was horrified to learn that the simple test is typically not done until a woman has three miscarriages. *Why*, she agonizingly wondered, *would the medical community let you endure multiple pregnancy losses before looking for a solution?* Although she grieved losing her second child as well, she was grateful her doctor had at least investigated for this condition before a third miscarriage. Once APS was her diagnosis, as soon as she got pregnant for a third time she was immediately given daily injections of a blood thinner. As the pregnancy progressed, those injections increased to twice a day. She needed to deliver two weeks early, but she finally experienced the joy of a live birth after the devastation of a repeat miscarriage.

To learn more about what ethical options are available for couples who face infertility, consider the work of NeoFertility, a cutting-edge fertility clinic in Dublin, Ireland, that has a higher pregnancy success rate than IVF. As they report on their website, "According to the HFEA [Human Fertilization and Embryology Authority], in 2017 the simple live birth rate for IVF was 26.4%. NeoFertility's average live birth rate for all patients who complete the programme is 53.6%." What is key about NeoFertility's approach is that they identify and address the underlying reason(s) for infertility, rather than pursue IVF, which really overlooks a problem. By correcting the reason for infertility at its origins, they help couples so that when they have sexual intimacy, they are more likely to get pregnant. For example, through NeoFertility's treatment of couples who had three or more miscarriages, 80 percent of them, according to 2010 statistics, had successful pregnancies.

Some women have difficulty conceiving because they have a problem referred to as low anti-Müllerian hormone (AMH) levels, or diminished ovarian reserve. Using ultrasound to track the maturation of a woman's ovarian follicle, timed blood tests, and training in fertility tracking, NeoFertility has helped women facing this condition achieve a successful pregnancy. They report, "The lowest AMH blood result we have achieved success with was for a 36 year old woman with 6 years of infertility who never conceived previously—her AMH was only 0.07 pmol/l (0.009 ng/dl) and her FSH was 42 iu/l. She conceived on her first cycle of treatment in our program and delivered a 9lb baby boy."

A lot of women face endometriosis, which can cause infertility. But IVF does not have to be the response to this condition either. My friend Sadie was diagnosed with endometriosis and had surgery. Four years later, she had a baby. Indeed, interventions can include laparoscopy so that endometriotic lesions are excised. NeoFertility treats endometriosis and other causes of infertility with great success, and all the while maintains respect for the sacredness of the sexual union of the couple. In other words, they assist an act of intercourse in achieving its end of pregnancy without substituting for sex. By working to correct pathologies in the woman or man and helping the body to function in optimal condition, a couple is more likely to achieve pregnancy without involving external parties in the heart of their one-flesh union.

The positive track record of NeoFertility even includes pregnancy in the face of a common condition that can result in infertility: polycystic ovary syndrome (PCOS), which is a hormonal disorder. One of the moving testimonies they share is of one of their patients who had three successful pregnancies even though she had PCOS.

My friend Claire from chapter 1 had successful surgery to treat PCOS. She traveled from her home state to Virginia just to get the help of a surgeon who was a specialist in ovarian wedge resection. The doctor had told her that due to many cysts, eggs weren't releasing because the cystic environment made for a type of leathery skin on her ovaries. The physician therefore advised that trying to force eggs out with hormone treatment likely would not be effective in that hostile environment. Instead, she proposed a surgery whereby she cut out a wedge from each ovary (the most cystic portions) and reattached the sides of the ovary together. This thinned out the skin so things could be absorbed and released as they are designed to be. This was highly specialized laparoscopy done with the assistance of a da Vinci robot.

For the next year, Claire and Jeremiah tried conceiving, but to no avail. Twelve months later, they returned to their surgeon in

Virginia and stayed for a week so that each day they could go to the clinic and have an ultrasound done to observe whether Claire's body was actually maturing a follicle and releasing an egg. As they witnessed on-screen, her body finally did what it was supposed to do (ovulate), and they were filled with joy and relief. But sexual intimacy that month *still* did not bring about conception.

The next month, however, on Jeremiah's birthday, Claire took a pregnancy test, and it was positive. She remembers being pregnant with that first child, sitting on their stairs with her ever-expanding bump, crying; she was so moved thinking about how hard they had worked to get there. Moreover, she realized at that moment that although she was nearing the end of her pregnancy, no matter how much work they had done, she was still not in control. She said, "I don't get to decide if I make it to birth with a healthy baby. It's still a mystery." Her husband said, "In every phase of your life, no matter what you're going through, there's plenty of suffering and sacrifice and yet still plenty of things to enjoy and rejoice about. I think we forgot to rejoice in the things we had to rejoice in. We were very focused on the suffering and sacrifice and that's where the tension came from. We weren't enjoying each other as we should have because we were too focused on the suffering."

Approaches like the surgery Claire had, or the interventions of NeoFertility, are examples of what is called Restorative Reproductive Medicine (RRM). It is described as

> an approach to reproductive medicine that uses medical and surgical techniques to identify and correct underlying medical problems such as poor ovulation, inadequate hormones, or immune factors. It does not bypass reproductive health issues but

> seeks to normalize or optimize natural reproductive function for women and men. It often uses a cycle or fertility chart to identify and time tests and treatments. The result is not only healthy cycles and normal function, but healthy pregnancies. Unlike IVF that often produces multiple pregnancies or pregnancies that deliver early and with low birth weights, RRM babies are mostly singleton pregnancies with healthy birth weights born at term. This is likely due to correcting factors that lead to difficult pregnancies and to closely monitoring RRM pregnancies and supplementing hormonal deficiencies when identified.

The International Institute for Restorative Reproductive Medicine (IIRRM) is based in London and has board member physicians from around the world. These include Dr. Phil Boyle from NeoFertility in Ireland along with physicians from Canada and the United States (California, North Carolina, Utah, New York, New Jersey, Minnesota, Louisiana, and Wisconsin). Although IIRRM is not directly connected to any other organization, its website provides links to like-minded organizations in the United States, Europe, Australia, and Africa, giving hope to couples around the world for ethical solutions to infertility. Whether labeled as "RRM," the previously mentioned "NaProTechnology," or "Creighton," there is a growing body of evidence-based medicine that helps couples achieve pregnancy without recourse to IVF.

It is worth underscoring this point: because IVF has become so commonplace, because it is a money-making business, and because some people think it is easier to ignore an underlying problem rather than address it, remedies that address health problems at their root are often overlooked. It perhaps shouldn't be surprising, then, that even when couples have had a failed IVF attempt, some of them manage to achieve pregnancy naturally when they pursue a corrective path.

In 2018, *Frontiers in Medicine* published a research paper titled "Healthy Singleton Pregnancies From Restorative Reproductive Medicine (RRM) After Failed IVF." As the paper reveals in its results, "403 patients met the study criteria, among which 74 had a subsequent live birth. These women had significant negative predictive characteristics for healthy live birth including: advanced reproductive age (average 37.2 years), an average of 5.8 years of infertility with 2.1 (range 1–9) previous IVF attempts, with only 5% having previously had a live birth from IVF." When all odds seemed against getting pregnant (most significantly having had failed IVF rounds), some women nonetheless achieved pregnancy with the help of RRM.

While more attention should be given to ethical fertility centers that take the approach of RRM, it is a sad truth that not everyone who wants to get pregnant will actually achieve it. Some causes of infertility cannot be corrected. When a couple is unable to achieve the birth and raising of their own biological children, it doesn't mean they will never be parents. There are children in our own countries and around the world who are in need of temporary or forever homes, and the Scriptures clearly command us to "care for orphans" (James 1:27). Fostering and/or adoption can meet those children's needs. Doing so is yet another way to reweave *shalom* in our broken world: it brings restoration to orphans by giving them parents they so badly need and deserve. Couples who face infertility might be more inclined to adopt, but infertility in no way needs to be part of the criteria for pursuing adoption.

In fact, in my travels, I met an inspiring family who adopted two children when their first biological child was only one year old. They have since adopted two more children, both of whom have Down syndrome and serious heart conditions, along with having more biological kids. The mother, Brianna, wrote,

> When we adopted my sons, we went from being a family of three to a family of five. As one would expect, we got a lot of "Why are you doing that?" and, when I became pregnant four months after my sons joined our family (taking us to a family of six), a lot of "Was this an accident?" And when I answered no, a lot of dumbfounded looks. What struck me most back then (and still does today) is that people were incredulous not so much because of the number of children we had, but simply because we were saying yes. Being open. Allowing love to grow and exponentially multiply, which it always does when a family is graced with new life.
>
> Those early years of our marriage with four itty-bitty children were outright hilarious, but they were beautiful too. If I could go back for a time, I would. A three-year-old sister sneaking cookies from the pantry to distribute to two-year-old brothers. Sloppy kisses and chubby hands welcoming a new baby sister. Exhausted parents collapsing onto the couch at the day's end, laughing at how ridiculously amusing our life was.
>
> But there was love. Always.

Friends of mine struggled with infertility for just over four years. The wife shared with me that her husband had always been interested in adoption, as was she. Although they discovered infertility after the start of their marriage, their openness to adoption preceded that. Their plan was to experience parenting through having biological children first and then pursue adoption. But as the wife said, "Infertility just changed the order of how our family was created." They adopted several children and ended up eventually conceiving several of their own biological ones as well. The wife's advice for couples considering adoption was this: "I would encourage them to go for it. It has been a real blessing in my life. Life is messy; jump right in. There will never be the perfect time or the perfect child, but God makes perfection out of our brokenness, so pray about it and put your trust in God."

After failed infertility treatments, Mariam and Kenneth pursued adoption (which was an idea Mariam had actually journaled about at the tender age of ten). Their eyes were opened to a number of things. First, when visiting Mariam's extended family overseas, word spread about this young Canadian couple wanting to adopt. They were told there was a couple willing to get pregnant *for* them, for a cost of $5,000 up front, along with another $5,000 at birth. Mariam and Kenneth were horrified that people would essentially market and traffic human children. That was a rude awakening, and although not all international adoption is like that, they decided that when they did pursue adoption, they would do so domestically.

Even with that, however, they went into it with one perspective and came out with another. Originally, they wanted to sign up just for infants. They learned that children available for adoption through the provincial ministry were often older children whose stories typically involve being apprehended by the government because their biological homes were not safe. They took very helpful and eye-opening classes learning about fetal alcohol syndrome, withdrawal, drug addiction, and so forth. They were told, "These babies come with stories." Mariam and Kenneth realized that even when a couple has their own biological children, they have no guarantee what their child will be like or what challenges the child may face.

They discerned that they would be open to adopting older children. Their application was submitted, and as it should happen, nine months later they got a phone call. They said yes to the child in need; however, that adoption fell through (not on their end). Shortly after that, they got another call and were sent a two-hundred-page document detailing the story of a five-year-old girl in need of a forever home. Within two months, she became their daughter. When asked what the most beautiful thing about adoption is, Mariam responded, "You grow your family—it's the love you create as a family." Kenneth said, "The most beautiful thing is knowing your child is a gift." After a few years, they adopted domestically again, this time as a result of being connected to a university student who faced an unplanned pregnancy. Mariam and Kenneth speak of their two adopted daughters as being "real sisters" to each other and of the beauty of watching them grow up together. They love to share their stories of adoption because they are filled with joy and believe it can inspire others to consider the same.

My friends Bryan and Sadie pursued fostering, caring for two babies at two separate times. Sadie wrote,

> It was so rewarding to see how quickly these scared babies began to feel secure (really within a couple of days) and then just bathed in the security, affection, and structure that we provided them. Older children would take longer to settle in, but babies are

> so programmed to accept care. Couples and families shouldn't underestimate the gift that they are able to provide foster children. I remember an adult former foster child telling me how his time in foster care was the best time of his childhood. Things like having a clean bed and regular meals were amazing for him.

Although a rich season of safety and blessing can be provided to such children, short-term stays are not ideal. The changing environment is hard both for the foster child as well as the foster family (especially if there are other children in the foster home who will grieve the loss of departing children). As Bryan said, "It's difficult to see them go to another foster home. I would have rather seen them go to adoptive parents or adopt them ourselves. I shake my head at how often they move." The more children can be in a foster-to-adopt program, the better we reweave *shalom* for them by providing permanence and continuity of care.

Married love need not be sterile. Even if a couple does not pursue adoption or fostering, people can always focus on spiritual parenthood. Love, by nature, is fruitful, and a couple can look for ways that their love can bear fruit in the lives of people around them. They can draw out their spiritual maternity and paternity by being actively involved in the lives of their nieces and nephews, volunteering in the formation of children at their church, or signing up to be a mentor to a child from a broken home, to name a few ideas.

My friend Bethany, whose story is told in the next chapter, had infertility and is now beyond the age of conceiving. She is a Christian leader who travels the world helping people. She told me that her mom said to her one day, "You have more children than anyone I know." Bethany's reply? "It's because I have spiritual children, people who have come to faith through programs and youth work I've done around the world who may never know me by name but who have benefited from my fruitfulness." Moreover, there are a lot of young people in her life whom she nurtures and cares for. They may never see her as a mother or big sister figure, but she's invested in their well-being the way a mother would be. She's given them a part of who she is and has experienced this as a real honor. She said, "It's a beautiful privilege to love younger people, to call out the best in them, to be someone who spoils and honors them and sees their best. My husband and I get to be that for a lot of people. I love it when I take out my teenage young friends and I say, 'May I lay my hands on you and pray for you?' It's an honor to serve their needs." Bethany's international reach caused her to joyfully tell me, "I do work I could never do had I had children. It would be impossible if I had children."

This approach of spiritual parenthood, while bringing fulfillment, doesn't necessarily take away the pain of infertility; it doesn't take away the good desire to bear a child with one's spouse. I think of Maddy, whose story was told in chapter 1. She shared that her way of coping with infertility was severalfold. She said she was very open with God, telling him when she was upset: "Lamentation is a form of prayer," she told me. At the same time, she warned against becoming obsessed with having children: "I would tell people to always have hope, but at the same time don't let it consume your life. Don't become obsessed with it, making it a sole focus of your life. If we do that, then we forget there are other things God has for us."

She found it helpful to regularly write gratitude lists of all the blessings in her life. She also renounced, out loud, lies from Satan that threatened her peace. And she kept a note in her phone, which she continually added to, of the various ways God gave her signs of hope and messages for her to contemplate. For example, she is a teacher, and one day she had to teach her teenage students about women in the Old Testament who suffered from infertility. She was really anxious to address a topic that struck a chord with her personally. But during her lecture, one of the students asked, "I'm wondering why there were so many good people suffering with infertility. I think it's interesting that there are so many stories of people who couldn't have kids but then God gave them kids." The student's inquiry alone lifted Maddy's spirits, and she sensed God speaking to her through the exchange.

Maddy shared that without her faith, she could not imagine how she would have been able to handle her suffering. She candidly admitted to moments where she was angry at God, but then shared her belief that God would make something good come out of her suffering. "We may not understand it," she said. "But I believe it." Indeed, in John 9, Jesus' disciples see a man who had been blind since birth. They ask him, "Rabbi, who sinned, this man or his parents, that he was born blind?" Jesus answers, "Neither this man nor his parents sinned; he was born blind so that God's works might be revealed in him" (John 9:2–3).

Famous motivational speaker Nick Vujicic shares the impact that this passage had on him. He was born without arms and legs, and although he believes God has the power to give him limbs, God hasn't done that. And yet, he came to the realization that God's works are revealed every day through his life. Nick wows audiences around the world, spreads the Gospel, and has since gotten married and had four children, including twins. His positive outlook on life, amidst his disability, shows God's work in so many ways.

Carrying the cross of infertility is like any cross: some days are more difficult than others. And we cannot always understand why certain desires go unmet, so there is no denying that this can be a real suffering. At the same time, amidst our brokenness lies an opportunity for God to reweave *shalom*, for him to show his glory and to reveal his works. These might be shown through a cure, or they might be revealed through a transformation of our hearts. Either way, he does show his glory. In light of that, we could consider another blind man, Bartimaeus, who once cried out, "Let me see again" (Mark 10:51). We could let his words become our prayer: *Lord, let me see what you want. Lord, let me see the path you have for me. Lord, let me see your works revealed.*

13

Idols

I recall a time in my mid-to-late thirties when I lamented to my spiritual director about how I was still single after more than a decade of journaling to Jesus about my longing for a spouse. I expressed my deep desire for marriage and how frustrated I was that God had not blessed me with a husband. My spiritual director had journeyed with me for years and knew me in ways others did not; he therefore had the insight and authority to respond as he did. He gently but firmly challenged me with an accurate assessment of my heart: *he told me I had turned marriage into an idol.* He warned that if I did not allow my heart to be made right on this matter, then if I ever did get married, my false idol would only lead to heartache.

What is an idol? To answer that, we can go to the Scriptures where God gave Moses the Ten Commandments: "You shall have no other gods before me. You shall not make for yourself an idol, whether in the form of anything that is in heaven above, or that is on the earth beneath, or that is in the water under the earth. You shall not bow down to them or worship them; for I the LORD your God am a jealous God" (Exod. 20:3–5). Here God is conveying that he, and he alone, is to be worshiped. As songwriters Stuart Townend and Keith Getty wrote,

> In Christ alone my hope is found,
> He is my light, my strength, my song;
> This Cornerstone, this solid Ground,
> Firm through the fiercest drought and storm.
> What heights of love, what depths of peace,
> When fears are stilled, when strivings cease!
> My Comforter, my All in All,
> Here in the love of Christ I stand.

In other words, we are to find our fulfillment in Christ, and when we look to other things—even good things—for our fulfillment, it is as though we are bowing down to a false god. Because created things are not meant to satisfy like the Creator, we will eventually find ourselves disappointed and frustrated, possibly even hurting the object of our affection because that person knows, deep down, they are imperfect and incapable of fulfilling another the way God does. This is not to say that it is wrong to want good things or good relationships. Instead, it is to point out that when our unfulfilled desires for these result in us being miserable and brooding, even hostile toward God, then our desire has switched over to an idol.

As John Piper writes, "What is an idol? Well, it is the thing. It is the thing loved or the person loved more than God, wanted more than God, desired more than God, treasured more than God, enjoyed more than God. It could be a girlfriend. It could be good grades. It could be the approval of other people. It could be success in business. It could be sexual stimulation. It could be a hobby or a musical group that you are following or a sport or your immaculate yard."

In contrast to false idols, Abraham teaches us how we ought to place our loves, interests, and desires in subordination to God's ways—with trust and surrender, by believing without seeing. In the Scriptures, it says, "God tested Abraham" (Gen. 22:1). And how did he do that? He told him, "Take your son, your only son Isaac, whom you love, and go to the land of Moriah, and offer him there as a burnt offering on one of the mountains that I shall show you" (Gen. 22:2). Abraham obeyed; he was willing to submit to God's ways, even if that meant giving up his beloved son. In this case, God didn't actually want Isaac sacrificed; instead, he wanted Abraham's *will* sacrificed. As the angel of the Lord said, "Do not lay your hand on the boy or do anything to him; for now I know that you fear God, since you have not withheld your son, your only son, from me" (Gen. 22:12).

But Abraham wasn't always this trusting. Earlier in Genesis, we read about Abraham's wife Sarah (at the time called Sarai) being barren and yet God promising him a son as an heir and descendants too numerous to count. Instead of trusting God to bring this about according to his ways, Abraham and Sarah took matters into their own hands, arranging for Abraham to have sex with Sarah's maid. But the resulting son, Ishmael, was not who God intended to be the heir.

God is all-powerful, and if he does not orchestrate things (even the impossible) as our hearts desire, or exactly when our hearts desire, then, rather than do wrong, we should surrender to him and trust, believing "that all things work together for good for those who love God, who are called according to his purpose" (Rom. 8:28). Letting go of our idols either sets our hearts right before the fulfillment of desire, or it prepares us for a different, but still life-giving, path God has for us.

And that brings to mind an email I sent to my friend Bethany while writing this book. She and her husband have been married for over twenty years and have never been able to conceive a child. I asked if she would be willing to share her experience, and I was struck by her reply to me:

> I don't think my story is that interesting. I don't think we have been through heartache. We wanted children but weren't desperate to get pregnant. There isn't a lot of grief in our souls so I am not sure if that's the story you are looking for. We actually feel blessed. Very early on we felt the Lord call out the idol of having children. Although a blessing to have children, if our life only had meaning or was fulfilling if we had them then we didn't trust the Lord for the life he would give us. Does that make sense? Sounds harsh but we didn't feel the grief when we dealt with our idol. Let me be clear, I don't think that dealing with the idol always means you don't grieve, but it did for us.

I responded by telling Bethany that I thought her story was actually *profoundly interesting* and incredibly relevant for this book. I believe she and her husband, through their lived experience, have tapped into a key truth that can enlighten us. And it is a truth that Bethany came to *before* realizing offspring would not be part of her story. She told me, "In my personal devotional life, I had been learning about idols and about how we put our hope in things outside of God, about how we trust in things outside of God, about how our idols manipulate our relationship with God, causing us to look at him as a cosmic wish-granter." Indeed, we humans can fall into the trap of thinking that if we pray hard enough for something that is good, then God will simply grant it. But that isn't always true.

In Romans 2:4 we are asked, "Do you not realize that God's kindness is meant to lead you to repentance?" That passage had a particular effect on Bethany. As she started to identify various idols in her life, such as her reputation, self-centeredness, etc., it led her to repentance while maintaining a vision of the kindness of God. She was given a grace to not land at either extreme of seeing God as a type of genie who grants wishes or as someone who is extremely harsh. Instead, she saw God as a loving father who is goodness and beauty, and who longs for her to experience freedom. As she pursued deeper intimacy with the Father, the Son, and the Holy Spirit, her love grew, her faith deepened, and she identified idols in her life that were actually hurting her. Her inner dialogue was not "I'm terrible and awful," but instead "God wants my good."

Bethany had come to this insight before she and her husband were worried they would not get pregnant. They knew it might take longer to conceive because she had only one fallopian tube, but they still thought it possible. Plus, she was young (in her late twenties) and they had time. When they were not successful at getting pregnant, she took Clomid, a fertility drug that induces ovulation so she would have eggs to be fertilized through sexual intimacy. But no child was conceived. Then they moved to a stronger drug, whereby she got injections to stimulate egg release. That, too, failed in helping them conceive children. Their prayer through the whole process was, "Lord, if this is your will, would you please give us children? If you want us to raise children, please give us children."

Lack of success in the interventions they pursued would cause some to move to the next step of IVF. This is where all that Bethany had previously learned about idols came to the forefront of her mind. She said,

> We realized that there's something inherently wrong with saying, "Having children is so important that I will go to any length to have them." It's like the big idol in my life showed up when I started to think that way. I realized I believe in a lie that my life will only be fulfilled if I have children. I'm believing a lie that my life is significant if I'm a mother. I'm believing a lie that as a woman you can't have a full life without children. I just realized they were all lies. When I came to that epiphany, I started reading books by women . . . [and] came to learn that there were people *with* children who had made their kids into idols, and how that played out.

God opened up her eyes, and she sensed him saying to her, "I have plans for you Bethany, but I want to free you from your idols so you can live the fullest life I have possible for you."

And then her prayer of surrender came. She was able to say, "I really want children; I want to give children to my husband; I really want that; in fact, I *long* to do that. But if I can't, I don't want it to ruin the rest of my life. I will not blame you, God, and I will not be disappointed in you."

It was that transformation of her heart, the reweaving of *shalom*, the establishment of *spiritual* wholeness that allowed her to tell me,

"Do I feel sad I never had kids? Of course I would have loved to have children, but I've never grieved super deeply. I never felt that was my journey because God has given me more than I've ever expected. I've had more joy and fulfillment and purpose. I just feel in every way God's faithfulness and his kindness to me. I harbor no resentment toward him. We are blessed beyond belief." Certainly not everyone who longs for a child has turned their desire into an idol, but where that temptation may exist for some, Bethany's experience of surrender and trust offers us wisdom.

When I was thirty-four, I got engaged, but I never married that man because we broke up. Over the next several years, I struggled deeply with times of anger and bitterness toward God (unjustly so). Through that season of working through having made marriage an idol, God did much to transform my heart in his refiner's fire. One day, my brother-in-law gave me a little devotional in which the reader goes through reflections, imagining Jesus taking over handling all the burdens, worries, and fears one has. Then you pray, "O Jesus, I surrender myself to you; take care of everything!" Those words and reflections became a guiding light for me over the following years as my heart and mind were being made new.

During that period, on a couple of occasions, my spiritual director also encouraged me to write my deepest desires on paper and then light a match and burn them as a type of burnt offering to God. These were not actions to rid me of want but to rid me of idols. They were designed to free my heart from unhealthy attachments and from putting my desires ahead of God, so as to orient me to surrender to God's authority much like Abraham did with Isaac. (And God's plans very much *may* be our plans; however, as a friend of mine likes to say, "At his pace, with his grace.") Prayer and counsel were also part of my story during those years. And it's not like I could identify one moment where I changed from embracing an idol to embracing surrender and trust. Honestly, it's more like the moments came and went. There were highs and lows. But gradually, time after time, the Holy Spirit was shaping and reshaping, carving and pruning my heart. We don't always feel changed—until a new challenge comes.

I was to experience that in the fall of 2020, when, after finally marrying, my husband and I miscarried our first child, LaeLae. Friends and family would check in to ask how I was doing, and I would remark that I felt supernatural grace. I felt carried. I realized my heart had changed. Unlike past sufferings where I experienced deep frustration with God and blamed him, even with the loss of a baby I loved so deeply, had celebrated so publicly, and wanted so badly, I felt only sorrow and grief—but was free from any bitterness and anger. A friend wrote my husband and me a letter expressing sympathy, and then she mentioned that she prayed our hearts would not turn bitter toward the Lord. She shared a quote by Elisabeth Elliot that I found deeply moving: "The secret is *Christ* in *me*, not me in a different set of circumstances."

Elisabeth's words are powerful, but so is her story. She was a Christian missionary with her husband, who was speared to death by tribesmen in Ecuador. With deep faith and courage and as a young widow with a toddler, she moved into the jungle to share the Gospel with the very people who had taken the life of her beloved. She wrote, "The deepest things that I have learned in my own life have come from the deepest suffering. And out of the deepest waters and the hottest fires have come the deepest things I know about God." Her witness reminds me of Job's response to suffering: "The

Lord gave, and the Lord has taken away; blessed be the name of the Lord" (Job 1:21). Each time we say these words, we release the grip of idols on our hearts.

Letting go of our idols does not mean crushing good desires. After my first miscarriage and then a live birth, I had three more miscarriages in a row. I dearly wanted each of those children we lost, and that was understandably a good desire. Why my sweet ones died remains a mystery, as a myriad of medical tests turned up no explanation for my losses, and I was even taking progesterone to support those pregnancies. The many miscarriages did cause me to reflect on the fact that this earth is not our home. It has reminded me that my children are very much alive in the heaven that awaits me. It has reminded me that until our epic family reunion, my days are meant to be spent loving God and loving others better and better. It has taught me to live with an eternal perspective, to realize that the value of a child's life is in that life—not in its length. It has taught me that the worth of my children is in who they are as unrepeatable, irreplaceable individuals made in God's image; it is not based on how much time I get to spend with them on earth. My, and my children's, ultimate destination is heaven. How long we live on earth before getting there is not in my control. But loving life here until it reaches its destiny, however long or short that may be, is within my control.

So is it good to desire the existence of such little lives to love? Absolutely. And when we release our idols and live for God, are we meant to no longer desire the great good of children? Absolutely not. But what is important is that we maintain a rightly ordered perspective, be detached and surrendered, so that if our desires are not met, we nonetheless trust that God is good, even when our unmet desires cause us to not *feel* good.

Letting go of idols also does not mean that God will not fulfill our desires. In fact, I think of Maddy and Peter who, after years of struggling with infertility, had long given up on conceiving themselves but were shocked to find out that they were pregnant; they have since given birth to a baby girl. Indeed, letting go of our idols does not mean God will not fulfill our desires. His timing, however, is not necessarily ours. Sometimes his message is not "no," but rather "not yet."

Letting go of our idols also does not mean suppressing natural human emotions like sadness and disappointment. It is okay, and normal, to feel those things. What it means is grabbing hold of Christ and being content in him (and with him in us). It means clinging to him when we do not understand. It means making the desires of our hearts known and then surrendering them to his perfect will. It means trusting that God is good and has plans for our good.

This reminds me of the story of Horatio Spafford. He and his wife experienced much sorrow. In 1871, their young son died, and that same year, Horatio suffered a great loss to his business as a result of the Great Chicago Fire. Two years later, devastation would continue when his wife and four daughters sailed to the United Kingdom and their ship collided with another ship in the middle of the ocean. All four daughters died. When Horatio traveled across the sea to his surviving wife, it was on that journey, near the same spot where his precious children perished, that he composed the hymn we often sing today:

When peace like a river attendeth my way,
When sorrows like sea billows roll,
Whatever my lot, Thou hast taught me to say,
It is well, it is well with my soul.

Even though our bodies may be broken and on this earth may never be fixed, is it well with our souls? Because that, at the end of the day, is paramount.

14

Restoration and Healing

In light of all that has been said, some might be thinking about those who have already chosen IVF and those conceived by IVF. How ought we respond?

For the latter group, as mentioned earlier, people conceived by IVF bear the image of God just as those conceived naturally do. Although the circumstances of an IVF-conceived person's beginnings go against how God designed new life to be brought forth, that an unrepeatable, irreplaceable, willed-by-God individual now exists is proof of God "making all things new" (Rev. 21:5). God redeems all things and can take even our sins and draw good out of them. Children conceived by IVF are the great good that come from it. That does not make the original act good; rather, it means that God is all-powerful and can show his glory in any situation, writing straight with our crooked lines.

For those who have chosen IVF, the past cannot be undone. And so, one's IVF-related sins (e.g., creating children outside of sexual intimacy, endangering the lives of one's children, eugenic selection of one's children, freezing of one's children, experimentation on one's children, abandonment of one's children, killing one's children, and so forth) need to be confessed. These sins, like all sins, need to be laid at the foot of the cross. One must call on Jesus for mercy. The good news? That is why Jesus died and rose from the dead: *for our sins*. If we call Jesus our Savior, it is because we are admitting we need to be saved *from* something. It is freeing to identify what those things are.

Couples could pray over what names to give all the embryos they had created. Besides memorializing the children through named identities, couples could think about ways to remember the children, acknowledging that they did exist. If others are aware of one's past choice to do IVF, surrogacy, or sperm and egg donation/selling, a couple could share their new conviction that that was a mistake, so as to not lead anyone down the wrong path by example. Repentance, Christ's mercy, and healing can be one's new story. Psalm 51 can be the new cry of one's heart: "Have mercy on me, O God, according to your steadfast love; according to your abundant mercy blot out my transgressions. Wash me thoroughly from my iniquity, and cleanse me from my sin" (Ps. 51:1–2). One could take also these words to prayer:

> I will take you from the nations, and gather you from all the countries, and bring you into your own land. I will sprinkle clean water upon you, and you shall be clean from all your uncleannesses, and from all your idols I will cleanse you. A new heart I will give you, and a new spirit I will put within you; and I will remove from your body the heart of stone and give you a heart of flesh. I will put my spirit within you, and make you follow my statutes and be careful to observe my ordinances.

> Then you shall live in the land that I gave to your ancestors; and you shall be my people, and I will be your God. (Ezek. 36:24–28)

In short, one can respond to this new knowledge about the problems with IVF in these three ways: repent, remember, and remedy.

Conclusion

"I plan on being a grandmother."

My friend Bethany said that to me near the end of my interview. But how does someone who has never given birth and who never adopted become a grandma? Bethany elaborated,

> I met, by the grace of God, some people through a Christian ministry. Those friends never had children, but they met a young woman from overseas who immigrated to Canada. Because all her family was in Europe, they essentially spiritually adopted her. She eventually got married and had children and my friends consider her children their grandchildren. They live nearby; they go to the kids' sporting events; they are wholly integrated into each other's lives as if they were biological family. Because of them, I've been praying for grandchildren. And I believe God will give me grandchildren. I believe that I will be a grandma, not a blood grandma, but a grandma like my friend became.

Bethany's life, amid infertility, is filled with joy and hope. Her prayer and confidence are a reminder that our yearning for family, for children, and to see our children's children is stamped into our very being. We image God, after all, and God is a communion of persons. He created the family, and he loves creating. He is the Author of life, and describes it as "good" and even "very good" (Gen. 1:31).

So how does all that line up with putting restrictions on the creation of life, ruling out IVF? We would do well to remember these words from Isaiah 55:8: "For my thoughts are not your thoughts, nor are your ways my ways, says the LORD."

Our good desires, to be ethically fulfilled, must be guided by God's blueprint for how we were designed to flourish. Consider what the Twelve Steps (a recovery program developed by Alcoholics Anonymous) have in common with the Ten Commandments: both admit there is a power higher than ourselves. Bearing that in mind, creature should heed Creator, not out of fear but out of freedom. Just as IKEA's furniture designers give instructions for our benefit, just as car manufacturers tell us when a vehicle should receive diesel instead of gasoline to make it run properly, God's ways are meant for our flourishing.

That the human person should not be treated as an object for use is a principle that all people of goodwill embrace. That members of the human family are our equals and that we may not own one another leads to the conclusion that we may not mistreat fellow humans. IVF, no matter how good one's intentions, mistreats the youngest of our kind. By manufacturing children, it treats them as commodities, poisons the parent-child relationship, and can even lead to killing the most vulnerable. Beyond that, it enlists parties, external to one's marriage, to force into existence an unrepeatable and irreplaceable image-bearer whom our Creator designed instead to be *received* through the sacred—an act of exclusive sexual intimacy between spouses, a physical manifestation of their married love that images the communion of persons that is the Trinity.

Within the nature of being male or female, at the height of our maturity, is a call to fatherhood and motherhood. For some, that will be in physical form. For others, it will be in spiritual form. In all ways, our fulfillment of this most mature form should conform to *shalom*, to wholeness—as our Intelligent Designer intended.

In the epilogue scene of the musical *Les Misérables*, we hear, "To love another person is to see the face of God." Although humans are not God, we are set apart from the rest of creation by bearing his image. The sacred is also within us. We are temples of the Holy Spirit and ought to have a sense of awe, reverence, and respect—not only for the other but for the very way that temple was designed to come into being.

APPENDIX I

What to Do with Frozen Embryos?

Going forward, what should be done? Most obviously, there should be *an immediate stop* to all IVF and related unethical reproductive technologies (e.g., surrogacy, egg and sperm selling/donation) that manufacture human persons. No more human embryos should be intentionally created outside of marital sexual intimacy. Admittedly, in the current cultural climate, this is an ambitious goal. Because a lot would need to change politically and socially to achieve this, there are some practical approaches we can take in the meantime. This book is an important starting place, and bringing its content into conversations with others can help move public opinion. Sharing information about the alternatives to IVF is another important step. So is lobbying one's political representatives, as well as encouraging one's religious leaders to educate their communities and provide programs of healing.

In the course of these conversations, some might then ask, "What do we do with the embryos who have already been created and who are left suspended in a frozen state?" Because this book aims to address the most pressing issue, it takes the position that IVF should *not* occur instead of doing a deep dive into what to do after IVF *does* occur. But as for the latter question, identifying the most ethical response can actually be quite challenging. That's because when we go down the path of moral error, the further we depart from truth, the more difficult it becomes to correct the problem in a way that doesn't create *more* moral error. That leaves us where we are today, where ethicists and theologians are examining and debating the most ethical solution to this situation of injustice for these littlest humans among us. The ethical complexities could fill a whole other book. This appendix is included just to give you a sense of how challenging it is to identify the best response to our world's reality.

Consider the following: Some might suggest that since we adopt born children in need, it would be ethical to adopt preborn children in need too. On the surface, that seems like a great response. But challenges arise. Who, for example, would be candidates to adopt frozen embryos? Ideally, children should be raised by a father and mother, so some might suggest married couples. But if a married couple adopts a frozen embryo, the woman's womb is occupied for nine months by someone else's child. In a sense, they "close the womb" to conceiving their own offspring at that time. Is that ethical? Do couples have a responsibility to receive offspring God may want to bless them with who would only be created by an act of sex that would occur in the nine months the unrelated embryo would be there (*if* that embryo weren't there)? Moreover, could there be health consequences for a woman who rescues a frozen embryo (refer to chapter 8) that prevent her from having her own children in the future? What are the ethical implications of that?

Some might propose that couples who have infertility that is not correctable could be ethical candidates for embryo adoption because they aren't closing the womb to their own children, since their own conceptions are not a biological possibility. People might say that if a woman can be a wet nurse and provide breastmilk for a child who isn't her own, couldn't a woman be an embryo adopter and provide the nourishment and environment of the uterus for a child who is not her own? After all, some might argue, if creating a child outside of sex is a sin, then that sin is over. Isn't transferring the already existing child into your body like adopting a born child who was conceived in sin (e.g., through a hookup, rape, etc.)?

I know a couple who did this. They could not conceive their own children and truly wanted to rescue frozen embryos for the good of those children. When they went to the embryo adoption clinic, they were willing to accept whatever children were in need, regardless of disability or how long they had been frozen. Moreover, they wanted to adopt a sibling set in order to rescue multiple children and to keep siblings together.

A sibling set of ten embryos who had been frozen for more than a decade was in need, and they adopted all of them. They went through several rounds of insertions at separate times (to ensure that there weren't too many embryos in any given pregnancy). Sadly, most of the embryos miscarried. But when the husband and wife attempted a final rescue of the ninth and tenth children, those fraternal twins implanted successfully and were born. The wife acknowledged that how her adopted children came to be should not have happened. She firmly believes it was wrong they were created by IVF, but she is also grateful to have been able to rescue them from abandonment in a freezer.

Some might find this laudable. Others might struggle in their response—both acknowledging that this couple truly tried to rescue the children as ethically as possible while expressing concern that there is an important difference between adopting a born child and adopting a preborn child—namely, that by God's designs, a preborn child should only get into a woman's body by way of sex between spouses. With embryo adoption, however, we are using a third party to place a child in a woman's body—a child who would never have been able to get there through the marriage bed. Is the conception of a child so closely linked to the gestation of a child that it should be treated differently from the post-birth raising of a child?

Some might suggest that single women could be candidates for what could be called embryo fostering. They would suggest it is not surrogacy because that is about offering your body to meet the desires of born people, whereas embryo fostering (or adoption) would be offering your body to meet the needs of abandoned preborn children. Then that single woman could either raise the child herself or place the child for adoption after birth.

This has its own problems too. If such a single woman does not raise the child, then what about the emotional, psychological, and physical ramifications? Even if someone fosters a born child, it is important to recognize that, ideally, children would not be in temporary homes; they would be in permanent ones with a forever family. Fostering the born should be viewed as a last resort when children are not legally able to be adopted yet or do not have a forever home to go to. But with fostering preborn children, we would be prioritizing a less-than-ideal situation of a temporary home for a child rather than pursuing a permanent family from the beginning when that is legally possible.

Moreover, if a single woman were to pursue this, what if that negatively impacted her own ability to have children in the future?

What of the psychological toll this could have on her due to the strong physiological bond between her and the child that pregnancy brings about? What about the aspect of scandal: Could such an approach normalize out-of-wedlock pregnancies? Or would it provide a teaching opportunity about the dignity of preborn lives and the importance of helping them? And what of the aspect of fatherless children? Much research has been done on the harm children suffer who are not raised by a mother *and* a father.

Others would point out that even having the option of embryo adoption makes for an easy out for biological parents who intentionally created children and therefore have a responsibility to care for them. Katy Faust from Them Before Us writes,

> The only option that honors the rights of frozen children is not listed on the ASRM [American Society for Reproductive Medicine] website. These babies are not commodities to be swapped and traded, thawed and discarded, used for research, or donated to another family.
>
> They are the very real children of the mother and father who created them. They have the right to be implanted into their mother's womb and allowed to grow or terminate naturally like every other human prior to these "advances" in medical technology.
>
> Yes, that means some parents will have more children than they originally wanted. Yes, that means adults spending more than they planned to spend. But that's what responsible parenthood demands.
>
> Even in the non-IVF world, sometimes you don't get to plan your family. Sometimes your family plans you. When

> people make babies the old-fashioned way and abandon them, we rightly call them deadbeat parents. Only in donor-conception do we permit and celebrate parents discarding or donating their parental duties.

Should there be a mandate, then, that biological parents have a duty to return for their frozen embryos, no matter how many they intentionally created? This isn't without concern either. Those who morally object to a third party inserting embryos in a woman's body would say that that is still required to rescue one's own children, and therefore it is problematic. Beyond that, however, there are other complicating factors: What if the biological mother is dead? What if she had a hysterectomy? What if she went through menopause? It gets even more complicated: Some embryos created and frozen were made using the gametes of people who have never been in a relationship with each other (sperm and egg sellers/donors). Who is morally responsible for the subsequent child? The parents who commissioned the child's creation? The woman whose egg was used to create the child? The man whose sperm was used to create the child? Or what about couples who created and froze embryos while together but then separated or divorced?

That's the story of actress Sofía Vergara and her now ex-fiancé Nick Loeb. They created two frozen embryos and have been in court battles. The media reports that Vergara wants them frozen indefinitely, whereas Loeb wants full custody to bring them to term. Even if Loeb succeeds in getting custody, he is incapable of gestating his own children. If he hires a surrogate, that would create another immoral step in an already messy situation.

Others might say that if we cannot ethically keep someone alive, then letting someone die is morally acceptable since death is ultimately a part of life, and not being able to save someone is very different from killing. For example, imagine that an unethical scientist manages to create embryos in a lab and gestate them in artificial wombs for nine months. (Yes, this is a futuristic, sci-fi scenario, but it is a thought experiment that will help us understand a point.) Imagine the scientist is doing an experiment where he intentionally creates humans who will need kidneys with the plan of transplanting lab-made kidneys when the lab-made humans are born. Imagine the scientist fails at successfully developing lab-made kidneys but has a large group of lab-made infants who will die without kidneys. Then imagine his lab is raided, and all these sick children are discovered. Without lab-made kidneys, imagine the only way to save the infants would be to give them transplants from other infant humans. But it is not ethical to make a born child be a kidney donor without his or her consent. Although people can survive with one kidney, it is still optimal to have two. So although "technically" there are born infants with kidneys that could be used to help these sick infants, it would not be moral to pursue their involvement.

Therefore, in the absence of an ethical option to save the lab-made children, wouldn't we acknowledge that how they were created to begin with was wrong, and give them comfort and care just as someone at the end of life would get in palliative care or hospice until they die naturally?

Would we likewise say that the uterus of a woman is not for just any children, except those of her and her husband, and that a freezer is not an environment keeping with the dignity of a human child?

As a result of there being no ethical place for the orphan embryos, would we, depending on denominational standards, baptize or dedicate them and ultimately give them a Christian burial?

Others might suggest we keep the embryos frozen until Christ's Second Coming. Some might reply that that approach would be not only an excessive cost when we do not plan on ever thawing them but also an ongoing injustice to the frozen embryos. They might point out that by keeping the embryos frozen, they are both denied the chance to grow up as well as the chance of more immediate eternal life (because who knows when the end of the world will actually happen).

As the points above make clear, when people discuss how to respond to the reality of frozen embryos, there are a lot of weighty matters to consider. But even as people weigh the pros and cons of these various responses, we first need to acknowledge that IVF is unethical to begin with, that it should not have been pursued and should no longer be pursued. As ethicists debate about how to respond to the morally messy situation that the pursuit of IVF created, what we need now is the wisdom of Solomon, who asked God to "give your servant therefore an understanding mind to govern your people, able to discern between good and evil" (1 Kings 3:9).

APPENDIX 2

Summary of Questions from This Book

Throughout his public ministry, Jesus employed the art of asking questions when conversing with others. This "Socratic" approach (named after the Greek philosopher Socrates) is powerful because it provokes deep thought. A question invites the questioned to consider what explanations and reasons they have for claims they or others make. It draws out critical thinking and helps us process in order to go beyond the surface of something.

There were various questions presented in this book, and here is a selection of them for further thought and reflection.

Introduction

1. Is it ethical to create human beings by science and not by sex?

Chapter 1

1. Do we have a right to demand a child?
2. Why is slavery wrong?

3. If we do not have a right to a fellow human, how should we view each other?
4. If one human may not possess another, then who possesses a human?
5. Although a woman may view her surrogacy as gift-giving, and therefore has good motives and not malicious intentions, is it her gift to give?

Chapter 5

1. What will be the fate of the remaining children created by IVF?
2. Is it ethical to endanger the lives of some children in an effort to create other children?
3. What if all embryos inserted implant? What if some or all of them become identical twins?

Chapter 7

1. Does having better intentions than someone else, by itself, make an action moral?

Chapter 8

1. What happens if a child is less than "perfect"?
2. We donate clothes to a thrift store; we donate paintings to a museum; but how is it ethical to "donate" a fellow human we ought not to own?
3. If a slave owner decided to "donate" his slave to another plantation, wouldn't we be just as outraged as if he sold that slave? Wouldn't we acknowledge that either approach treats

the slave—a human being—as though she is a possession owned by someone else?

4. Should the creative capacity of human beings—both the personal life-giving potential in our gametes as well as the offspring we are parents of—ever be treated like a business?

Chapter 10

1. Does it fit with God's designs about sexual intimacy to enlist a third party, outside of a married couple, when it comes to the very moment of creating new life?

Chapter 11

1. Is it possible that, as we have lost the sense of the sacred in the temple of our church buildings and worship, we have correspondingly lost the sense of the sacred in the temple of our bodies?
2. We are meant to have great reverence when handling and interacting with the human body. That is why we have a duty to bury the dead and have laws against mistreating corpses. If that is our responsibility to a body that has no life, then how much more of a responsibility do we have for the body that is very much alive?

Chapter 13

1. What is an idol? Can pregnancy, parenthood, and children become idols? How can we free ourselves from this?

APPENDIX 3

Responding to Common Objections

Having read this far, your mind is likely swirling with a lot of information. Now the challenge is this: How do you share the content of this book in conversation with others? What follows are some common questions people might ask, along with brief responses, and then a reminder of the relevant chapters you can return to for further details.

Infertility is a sign of the body not working properly. Shouldn't we be willing to help people correct this problem?

It is absolutely reasonable to want to fix problems. No one is objecting to that. Instead, what is being questioned is the *means* used to correct problems. After all, don't we agree that kidnapping is not an ethical solution to fulfilling one's desire for children? That is an example of a reasonable desire corrected in a morally problematic way. Similarly, there can be other "solutions" to the problem of infertility that are not ethical. For more information, go to chapters 3 and 9. Having said that, there are plenty of ethical solutions to the problem of infertility. Review chapter 12 for examples.

If someone is critical of IVF, it sure sounds like they are being critical of the very individuals who were created that way. Without IVF, some people would not exist.

It is true that someone conceived by IVF would not exist had that procedure not happened. And yet, there are a lot of humans who would not exist if the circumstances of their conception did not happen either. People who hook up but have no love for each other may create a baby. Such lustful use of another is not moral, and yet the individual child who comes to be as a result of that is still unrepeatable, irreplaceable, and unique. Don't we separate actions from actors all the time? For example, parents who discipline their children for doing something wrong aim to convey that they *love their child* but they *do not love the bad behavior of the child*. Likewise, if we believe all humans are equal, then isn't it possible to see the dignity and value in each person who is conceived while not validating all the ways someone may come into existence (for example, lust or even violence)? Turn to chapters 3 and 14.

Don't people have a right to have children?

Imagine a couple who lives in a country where the government limits the number of children they can have. That would be unjust. In that context, a couple could rightly reply, "We have a right to be open to as many children as God blesses us with." But that right does not give them license to manufacture humans; instead, it gives them protections from governments stopping their intimate sexual act from achieving its natural end of offspring. In other words, governments do not have a right to limit the freedom of individuals to be open to what could naturally flow from marital intimacy. At the same time, a couple may not demand the government *make them* children. Any offspring that come about should be received as a *gift* from God the Creator, rather than as an object to be manufactured. We do not have a right to demand a gift from God or force an individual into existence. Since a child is a human being who is a subject and not an object, we should not view a human as a possession. See chapter 4.

Scientists just want to use their talent and knowledge to help people.

It is good to put our gifts at the service of others. Isn't it important, though, to ensure that we are actually helping and not hurting people in the process? IVF involves harming and even killing some of the tiniest humans among us. It also treats both the preborn and the born as commodities. There are examples throughout history of people in the medical and scientific fields who made decisions to help one person at the expense of others, and now we look back at that in horror. Review chapters 4, 5, and 8.

In objecting to IVF, it sounds like you are against things that use technology. But isn't implanting a pacemaker using technology? If that is acceptable, then why isn't IVF?

As you rightly point out, there are various medical interventions that are morally acceptable that use technology. The problem with IVF is that it goes against God's designs for how humans were meant to come into existence: it manufactures someone who is not an object. In doing so, it intentionally makes and places some humans in an environment that is unsafe and could lead to their harm or death, all in an effort to make other humans. It is worth considering that there is a difference between parts and wholes. For example, if your heart isn't working optimally, by using a pacemaker you are restoring the body part to its proper function. The same could be said for our reproductive organs that are not working properly: it is acceptable to use technology to, for example, unblock fallopian tubes so that eggs, sperm, and embryos can pass through as designed. But IVF is different. It is not about restoring a body part to its proper function. It is about manufacturing into existence a whole person (and harming some persons in the process). In other words, the objection to IVF does not rest on being against progress or technology; instead, it rests on being opposed to exploitation and the twisting of the natural design of our relationships. There is a difference between preserving how a body part was meant to function and producing another human being entirely. See chapters 4, 10, 11, and 12.

God commanded us to be fruitful and multiply. Wouldn't IVF be a way to fulfill that command?

Just because IVF involves fruitfulness and multiplication, it does not logically follow that it is ethical. After all, promiscuity also yields those two things; yet would we say God endorses that? Instead, we should consider the command to be fruitful and multiply *within the context* of how God designed it to be fulfilled. Not only did God choose sex as the means for humans to reproduce, but he chose *marital* sex in particular. IVF does not require sex at all.

Moreover, it involves taking what comes in the most private and intimate of moments between a husband and wife—the climax of their lovemaking, which has the capacity to create new life—and outsources their offspring's beginning to an outside third party. See chapters 9, 10, and 11.

Even though there are problems with some ways of doing IVF, isn't it possible for it to be ethical within certain parameters, such as only using a husband's and wife's gametes? In other words, I see how it is wrong for strangers, but what about a loving, married couple?

Certainly a loving, married couple is in the right relationship that God designed for offspring. One of the problems with IVF, even in this context, is that it not only involves the married couple; it also outsources their offspring's beginning to scientists in a lab. Human beings are not products to be manufactured. Instead, we were meant to come to be as a result of a communion of persons between our parents, who then receive the gift of life, an ensouled human being whom God makes in his image. See chapters 9, 10, and the chart at the end of chapter 11.

What can ethically be done to help people who face infertility?

It is good to identify what is at the heart of someone's infertility. For example, do they have a hormone imbalance that can be regulated with a prescription? Do they have blocked fallopian tubes that can be repaired through surgery? By correcting the problem at its root, the body is not only restored to optimal health and functioning, but it is more likely to achieve pregnancy from sexual intercourse. With these types of interventions, a married couple's sexual acts are aided in achieving their proper end of offspring without actually replacing the sexual act itself or involving a third party to manufacture life. For specific examples of ethical interventions in response to infertility, see chapter 12. Having said that, in this broken world, not all sickness and imperfection can be corrected. That is where chapter 13's remarks on idols offer a helpful reflection.

If you had to summarize the reasons to object to IVF, what would they be?

IVF harms and kills some human beings. It involves practices that violate the nature of parenthood and the responsibility of mothers and fathers to ensure the safety and protection of their offspring. It also treats humans, both the preborn and the born, as commodities. More fundamentally, it divorces sex from the creation of life and replaces a married couple with a scientist when it comes to their child's beginning. In contrast to IVF, the Scriptures reveal how God designed a husband and wife to come together in a communion of persons, in a private and intimate act, to receive offspring as a gift rather than involve a third party to manufacture a child as a product. This last point often takes more fleshing out for people to grasp, and part 3 goes into it in depth.

Notes

INTRODUCTION

1 **In the documentary *Anonymous Father's Day*, viewers meet the man behind this story:** The Center for Bioethics and Culture Network, "*Anonymous Father's Day* (Full Film)," YouTube video, June 3, 2016, https://www.youtube.com/watch?v=fFd94VE--8g.

1 **Consider the Donor Sibling Registry website:** "History and Mission," Donor Sibling Registry, accessed October 3, 2024, https://donorsiblingregistry.com/history-and-mission.

1 **The largest group is two hundred half-siblings:** CBS Sunday Morning, "Sperm Donor Dad Bonds with the Kids He Never Knew He Had," YouTube video, January 10, 2016, https://www.youtube.com/watch?v=Il7HhOMpVQg.

2 **Fertility clinics could have sold as many as 9,600 vials:** CBS Sunday Morning, "Sperm Donor Dad."

3 **The Obamas' pursuit of IVF:** Michelle Obama revealed this in her memoir. See Michelle Obama, *Becoming* (New York: Crown, 2018), 187–190.

3 **Nicole Kidman's pursuit of IVF:** "Nicole Kidman Announces Baby Born through Surrogate," BBC News, January 18, 2011, https://www.bbc.com/news/entertainment-arts-12213615.

3 **Céline Dion's pursuit of IVF:** Danielle Fowler, "11 Celebrities Who Have Opened Up About Their IVF Experiences," *Marie Claire* (Australia edition), November 17, 2020, https://www.marieclaire.com.au/news/celebrity/celebrities-spoken-about-ivf.

3 Louise Brown became the first successful "test tube baby": Susan Scutti, "At Least 8 Million IVF Babies Born in 40 Years since Historic First," CNN, July 3, 2018, https://www.cnn.com/2018/07/03/health/worldwide-ivf-babies-born-study/index.html.

3 Five hundred thousand babies born annually as a result of IVF: "More Than 8 Million Babies Born from IVF since the World's First in 1978," ScienceDaily, July 3, 2018, https://www.sciencedaily.com/releases/2018/07/180703084127.htm.

3–4 "Unborn children are 'children' under the Act": LePage v. Center for Reproductive Medicine, SC-2022-0515.

4 Alabama legislators were quick to respond: Jemma Stephenson, "Alabama Senator Files Bill to Protect IVF Services in State; Hearings Set for Wednesday," Alabama Reflector, February 27, 2024, https://alabamareflector.com/2024/02/27/alabama-senator-files-bill-to-protect-ivf-services-in-state/.

4 Proposal that states that ban IVF access be denied Medicaid funding: "Sens. Cruz, Britt Introduce Legislation Protecting IVF," Ted Cruz (website), May 20, 2024, https://www.cruz.senate.gov/newsroom/press-releases/sens-cruz-britt-introduce-legislation-protecting-ivf.

5 Miscarriage risk climbs to roughly 40 percent at forty: Alexandra Benisek, "Pregnant at 40: What to Expect," WebMD, February 14, 2023, https://www.webmd.com/baby/pregnant-at-40.

PART I

CHAPTER I

9 Thirty-four million more men than women in China: Simon Denyer and Annie Gowen, "Too Many Men," *Washington Post*, April 18, 2018, https://www.washingtonpost.com/graphics/2018/world/too-many-men/.

10 Devastating effects of this gender imbalance: FRANCE 24 English, "Video: Millions of Single Chinese Men Desperately Seeking a Wife," YouTube video, June 9, 2017, https://www.youtube.com/watch?v=3b0N2luN6Nc.

10 "I feel like I'm invisible": FRANCE 24 English, "Millions of Single Chinese Men."

CHAPTER 2

18 "I have constantly asked myself: *What do I respect?*": Matthew Kelly, *Perfectly Yourself: 9 Lessons for Enduring Happiness* (New York: Ballantine, 2006), 63, 65, emphasis in the original.

18 Love as willing the other's good: *Catechism of the Catholic Church* 1766 quotes from St. Thomas Aquinas: "To love is to will the good of another."

CHAPTER 3

19 "My husband said to me: 'You are my slave'": Denyer and Gowen, "Too Many Men."

19 His family locked her in the home: Denyer and Gowen.

20 "Lansui paid her smugglers": FRANCE 24 English, "Millions of Single Chinese Men."

20 The dialect in her husband's village: "Millions of Single Chinese Men."

21 I unpack in other writings: See *My Body for You: A Pro-Life Message for a Post-Roe World* (Steubenville, OH: Emmaus Road, 2023).

CHAPTER 4

26 "It is the most beautiful gift you could ever give": Teresa Woodard, "Surrogate Mother Who Refused Abortion Launches Effort to Change Laws," KHOU, December 21, 2018, https://www.khou.com/article/news/health/surrogate-mother-who-refused-abortion-launches-effort-to-change-laws/285-624461486.

26 "So she's writing a book about joy": Woodard, "Surrogate Mother."

PART 2

CHAPTER 5

31 "Most couples have at least three to five more embryos frozen": "What Happens to Stored Embryos if I Decide Not to Use Them?" Reproductive Resource Center, accessed October 3, 2024, https://www.rrc.com/what-happens-to-stored-embryos-if-i-decide-not-to-use-them/.

31 A procedure called ICSI: Hang With The Bangs, "IVF Fertilization Report," YouTube video, February 3, 2019, https://www.youtube.com/watch?v=9hmTu5sq6xU.

31–32 Of the remaining embryos, five were "really good": Hang With the Bangs, "IVF Embryo Transfer—Put a Baby in Me!" YouTube video, February 5, 2019, https://www.youtube.com/watch?v=t8s2K8rptNs&t=.

32 A total of five were frozen: Kelsey Bang, "Our IVF Twin Success Story," Kelsey Bang (website), May 6, 2020, https://kelseybang.com/2020/05/our-ivf-twin-success-story.html.

32–33 She should have been in university, not a nursery: Anna Hecker, "What Should I Do with My Unused Embryos?" *New York Times*, April 15, 2020, https://www.nytimes.com/2020/04/15/parenting/fertility/ivf-unused-frozen-eggs.html.

33 "80 to 90 per cent of embryos survive the thawing process": Sonya Kashyap, "Embryo Freezing vs. Egg Freezing: What You Need To Know," HuffPost, April 30, 2015, http://www.huffingtonpost.ca/dr-sonya-kashyap-md-msc-epi-frcsc-facog/frozen-embryos_b_7182806.html.

33 "Approximately 95% of embryos typically will survive the freeze-thaw process": "FET (Frozen Embryo Transfer)," Utah Fertility Center, accessed June 12, 2021, https://www.utahfertility.com/treatmentivf/advanced-techniques-ivf/fet-frozen-embryo-transfer/.

33 2.3 million embryos were discarded for the 1.7 million embryos transferred: "Embryos: Question for Department of Health," UK Parliament (website), November 22, 2016, https://questions-statements.parliament.uk/written-questions/detail/2016-11-08/HL3075.

33 The United States has one million human beings in freezers: "What We Do," National Embryo Donation Center, accessed October 3, 2024, https://www.embryodonation.org/.

34 **It seems the other sixteen did not succeed in implanting:** "How Do I Decide How Many Embryos to Transfer?" Dominion Fertility, October 25, 2011, https://www.dominionfertility.com/blog/50-how-do-i-decide-how-many-embryos-to-transfer.

34 **"If multiple pregnancies occur, a multifetal selective reduction can be considered":** "How Do I Decide How May Embryos to Transfer?"

35 **"Some people prefer to dispose of their embryos":** "Embryo Freezing," Human Fertilisation & Embryology Authority, accessed October 3, 2024, https://www.hfea.gov.uk/treatments/fertility-preservation/embryo-freezing/, emphasis added.

35 **"To become destroyed or ruined: cease to exist":** *Merriam-Webster*, s.v. "perish," last modified September 15, 2024, https://www.merriam-webster.com/dictionary/perish.

CHAPTER 6

36 **"We have the same hair and we have the same eyes":** The Center for Bioethics and Culture Network, "Breeders: A Subclass of Women," YouTube video, July 20, 2021, https://www.youtube.com/watch?v=rA0J1HH2gZw.

38 **"I can't help but think 'This is my sister' every time I look at her now":** Emily Yoffe, "My Wife Is My Sister," Slate, February 19, 2013, https://slate.com/human-interest/2013/02/dear-prudence-my-wife-and-i-came-from-the-same-sperm-donor.html.

38 **"Do *I* matter?":** Elise Hilton, "A Marketplace of Children: The Fertility Industry," Acton Institute, May 29, 2014, https://blog.acton.org/archives/69240-marketplace-children-fertility-industry.html.

38 **The impact that had on the mind of eight-year-old Alana:** As told in the documentary *Anonymous Father's Day*. See The Center for Bioethics and Culture Network, "Anonymous Father's Day (Full Film)," YouTube video, June 3, 2016, https://www.youtube.com/watch?v=fFd94VE--8g.

38 **"Newman describes this as the man's 'symmetrical' relationship":** Emma O'Friel, "Donor-Conceived Adults: A Lifelong Search for Identity," *Irish Times*, July 22, 2017, https://www.irishtimes.com/life-and-style/health-family/parenting/donor-conceived-adults-a-lifelong-search-for-identity-1.3161451.

39 **"I wish I even knew how to describe how wonderful and awful it has been":** "Silently Longing," Anonymous Us Project, December 5, 2019, https://anonymousus.org/silently-longing/.

39–40 "I have an abusive single mother who bought me to fill her loneliness": "Dear Current and Prospective Parents, Please Read This," Anonymous Us Project, March 27, 2019, https://anonymousus.org/dear-current-and-prospective-parents-please-read-this/.

40 "Advance social policies that encourage adults to actively respect the rights of children": Katy Faust, "The White Paper—Who We Are and Why We Exist," Them Before Us, May 12, 2018, https://thembeforeus.com/white-paper/.

40–41 "Donor children struggle disproportionately with depression, delinquency, and substance abuse.": Katy Faust, "Dear NY, Commercial Surrogacy is Bad for Kids," Them Before Us, February 27, 2019, https://thembeforeus.com/dear-ny-commercial-surrogacy-is-bad-for-kids/.

CHAPTER 7

42 Left in cold freezers at temperatures as low as –320 degrees Fahrenheit: "Embryo Storage FAQs," ReproTech, accessed October 3, 2024, https://www.reprotech.com/embryo-storage-faqs/.

42 "Twenty-one percent of our embryos have been abandoned": Mary Pflum, "Nation's Fertility Clinics Struggle with a Growing Number of Abandoned Embryos," NBC News, August 12, 2019, https://www.nbcnews.com/health/features/nation-s-fertility-clinics-struggle-growing-number-abandoned-embryos-n1040806.

42–43 "A paper co-authored in the scientific journal *Nature Biotechnology*": Pflum, "Nation's Fertility Clinics."

43 "This technology allows doctors to select embryos": "PGD—PGD for Single Gene Defect," Reproductive Partners Medical Group, accessed October 3, 2024, https://www.reproductivepartners.com/southern-california-pgd.html.

43 "Orchid sequences over 99% of an embryo's DNA": "Home Page," Orchid Health, accessed October 3, 2024, https://www.orchidhealth.com/.

43–44 Proudly reveal how they can screen embryos for conditions: "Science," Orchid Health, accessed October 3, 2024, https://www.orchidhealth.com/science.

44 They can screen IVF-created embryos for more than 1,200 "single gene" conditions: "Science."

44 "Find the embryo at lowest risk for a disease that runs in your family": "Home Page," Orchid Health.

44 "When you conceive at home, random chance determines your child's genetics": "Orchid Guides Portal," Orchid Health, accessed October 3, 2024, https://portal.orchidhealth.com/risk-calculator.

44 "Based on the embryos' genetic health": "Orchid Guides Portal."

44 Willing to spend more than $12,000 getting a genetic profile: "Clinician Information," Orchid Health website, accessed October 3, 2024, https://www.orchidhealth.com/clinician-information.

45 "The Parents Who Want Daughters—and Daughters Only": Emi Nietfeld, "The Parents Who Want Daughters—and Daughters Only," Slate, May 7, 2024, https://slate.com/technology/2024/05/ivf-daughters-toxic-masculinity-sex-selection.html.

45 "Select the Gender and Eye Color of Your Next Baby": "Select the Gender and Eye Color of Your Next Baby," The Fertility Institutes, accessed October 3, 2024, https://www.fertility-docs.com/programs-and-services/gender-selection/select-the-gender-of-your-baby-using-pgd/.

45–46 "We've done it seven times. I have all boys": Angela Andaloro, "Paris Hilton Says She and Carter Reum Have 20 Boy Embryos Frozen and Are Still Trying for a Girl," *People*, February 26, 2023, https://people.com/parents/paris-hilton-20-boy-embryos-frozen-still-trying-for-girl/.

46 They welcomed the birth of a daughter, also via IVF and surrogacy: "Paris Hilton Announces the Arrival of a Baby Daughter, London," Associated Press, November 24, 2023, https://apnews.com/article/paris-hilton-baby-daughter-f1ebad6e792926cd0f8f69c883c4fe78.

46 "When I think about having a child that's a boy, it's almost a repulsion": Nietfeld, "The Parents Who Want Daughters—and Daughters Only."

46 "Embryos that possess a desirable genetic trait": "PGD—PGD for Single Gene Defect," Reproductive Partners Medical Group.

46–47 Two of their other children live in New York—as frozen embryos: Elissa Strauss, "The Leftover Embryo Crisis," *Elle*, September 29, 2017, https://www.elle.com/culture/a12445676/the-leftover-embryo-crisis/.

47 **"Embryos are useful":** Strauss, "The Leftover Embryo Crisis."

47–48 **An American surrogate shares her story of agreeing to gestate twins for a couple from Spain:** The Center for Bioethics and Culture Network, "*#BigFertility*," YouTube video, July 20, 2021, https://www.youtube.com/watch?v=QvQP7JSydMw.

48 **"We concluded that should our tides shift":** Strauss, "The Leftover Embryo Crisis."

48–49 **"In the bowels of Midtown Manhattan":** Hecker, "What Should I Do with My Unused Embryos?"

49 **"The highest expression of love has long been defined as a willingness to lay down your life":** "Opposites," Abort73, accessed October 3, 2024, http://abort73.com/videos/opposites/.

CHAPTER 8

51 **"During the IVF process, embryos created in the lab are graded":** "Embryo Grading: The Good, The Poor, and The Baby Making Kind," ORM Fertility, June 19, 2019, https://ormfertility.com/fertility/embryo-grading/.

52 **"Proud to be perfecting the use of elective single embryo transfer":** "Success Rates," Genesis Fertility & Reproductive Medicine, accessed June 12, 2021, http://genesis-fertility.com/about-us/success-rates/, emphasis added (site discontinued).

52 **Some IVF-conceived children with Down Syndrome were aborted:** Daniel Martin, "Dozens of IVF Babies Are Being Aborted Because They Have Down's syndrome," *Daily Mail*, July 15, 2012, http://www.dailymail.co.uk/health/article-2174068/Dozens-IVF-babies-aborted-Downs-syndrome.html.

52 **In the documentary *Breeders*, several women who chose to be surrogates tell their stories:** The Center for Bioethics and Culture Network, "Breeders: A Subclass of Women," YouTube video, July 20, 2021, https:// www.youtube.com/watch?v=rAoJ1HH2gZw.

52 **"You can donate your embryos to another woman with fertility problems":** "Frequently Asked Questions," Society for Assisted Reproductive Technology, accessed October 3, 2024, http://www.sart.org/patients/frequently-asked-questions/.

54 "You can donate your embryos for laboratory research": "Frequently Asked Questions."

54–55 "We have 2 collection rooms": "Guys Want to Know . . . What's in the Collection Room?" Michigan Reproductive Medicine, November 13, 2020, https://www.mireproductivemedicine.com/guys-want-to-knowwhats-in-the-collection-room/.

55–56 "If you are selected . . . you'll get $100 cash for each approved donation": "Earn Extra Money in 2022 as a Sperm Donor," Phoenix Sperm Bank, accessed October 3, 2024, https://www.phoenixspermbank.com/blog/earn-extra-money-this-year-as-a-sperm-donor/.

56 $8,000 to $10,000 *per* donation cycle: "How Much Money Do Egg Donors Get Paid?" Bright Expectations, June 29, 2018, https://www.brightexpectationsagency.com/blog/how-much-money-egg-donors-paid/.

56 "Egg donation is fundamentally altruistic": "Egg Donor Compensation," Bright Expectations, accessed October 3, 2024, https://www.brightexpectationsagency.com/egg-donor-compensation/.

56 "An intrinsically selfless decision": "Egg Donor Compensation."

56 "Based on generosity": "How Much Money Do Egg Donors Get Paid?"

57 Higher base if you're an "experienced" surrogate: "Surrogate Pricing & Costs," West Coast Surrogacy, accessed October 3, 2024, https://www.westcoastsurrogacy.com/surrogate-program-for-intended-parents/surrogate-mother-cost.

57 $10,000 to go ahead with destroying the child who was once desired: "Surrogate Pricing & Costs," accessed June 12, 2021.

57 She produced twenty eggs—almost two years' worth: Jane Ridley, "Being an Egg Donor Gave Me Terminal Cancer," *New York Post*, December 3, 2015, https://nypost.com/2015/12/03/being-an-egg-donor-gave-me-terminal-cancer/.

57 Breast cancer that had spread to other parts of her body: You can learn about Maggie Eastman in the documentary *Maggie's Story*. See The Center for Bioethics and Culture Network, "*Maggie's Story*," YouTube video, July 20, 2021, https://www.youtube.com/watch?v=jvaW6-oNJ9E.

57 "I feel like I was prostituted and kept in the dark about the possible toll on my health": Ridley, "Being an Egg Donor."

58 Her eggs may have been used to make untold numbers of humans: Ridley, "Being an Egg Donor."

58 "Revealed a statistically significant association between egg donation and onset of preeclampsia": Juan Enrique Schwarze et al., "Is the Risk of Preeclampsia Higher in Donor Oocyte Pregnancies? A Systematic Review and Meta-Analysis," *JBRA Assisted Reproduction* 22, no. 1 (March 2018): 15–19.

58 "The surrogate mother . . . think of her as an organ donor": "*#BigFertility.*"

58 Preeclampsia was the experience of a surrogate named Kelly Martinez: "*#BigFertility.*"

PART 3

CHAPTER 9

65–66 "Our sex cells, or gametes, are special cells": Tadeusz Pacholczyk, "Making Sense of Bioethics: Column 010: Sperm for Sale," The National Catholic Bioethics Center, April 30, 2006, https://www.ncbcenter.org/making-sense-of-bioethics-cms/column-010-sperm-for-sale.

66 "Hence, donating to sperm or egg banks violates something fundamental": Pacholczyk, "Making Sense of Bioethics."

CHAPTER 10

73–74 The man typically masturbates to provide a sperm sample: It is possible (although rare) for a man to use an alternative to masturbation: he could have sex with his wife using a special nontoxic condom in order to produce a sperm sample; however, to pursue IVF, the man nonetheless gives that collected semen to the IVF clinic rather than to his wife's body, and the child is still created at the hand of the scientist. Sexual intimacy is not being brought to its full completion with the possibility of conception in the wife's body but instead is interrupted to involve a third party in the moment of life's creation.

74 The assumed biological father was actually not her dad: "NJ Couple Sues Fertility Clinic, Saying Wrong Sperm Used to Conceive Child." ABC7 News, September 12, 2019, https://abc7news.com/fertility-clinic-mixup-new-jersey-lawsuit/5532537/.

74 The genetic offspring was mistakenly implanted in the wrong woman: "IVF: Second Couple Sue after Clinic 'Uses Wrong Embryos.'" BBC, July 11, 2019, https://www.bbc.com/news/world-us-canada-48948883.

74 More tragic stories like these from around the world: See, for example, Times of Israel Staff and Renee Ghert-Zand, "Parents of Baby Born in 2022 IVF Mix-up Found Through Testing," Times of Israel, March 7, 2024, https://www.timesofisrael.com/parents-of-baby-born-in-2022-ivf-mix-up-found-through-testing/; Hannah Ritchie, "Australian State Orders Sperm Bank Purge Over Mix-ups," BBC, July 2, 2024, https://www.bbc.com/news/articles/c4ngl45jz1zo; and Clare Dyer, "Biological Father Declared the Legal Father in IVF Mix Up," National Library of Medicine, March 8, 2003, https://www.ncbi.nlm.nih.gov/pmc/articles/PMC1169278/.

CHAPTER 11

82 Embryo is "begotten not made": This phrase, taken from the Nicene Creed, describes Jesus. Having said that, author C.S. Lewis explained this concept of being "begotten, not made" in his book *Mere Christianity* by saying, "When you beget, you beget something of the same kind as yourself. A man begets human babies, a beaver begets little beavers and a bird begets eggs which turn into little birds. But when you make, you make something of a different kind from yourself. A bird makes a nest, a beaver builds a dam, a man makes a wireless set" (C.S. Lewis, *Mere Christianity* [New York: HarperOne, 2001], 157). In this sense, a human child manufactured through IVF is "made"—the individual is different from the scientist who created him. Contrast that with a child conceived through sex who is begotten of the parents: the two individuals whose action brings offspring into existence are begetting someone who is their kin.

CHAPTER 12

84 "Natural Procreative Technology is a women's health science": "Home Page," NaProTechnology, accessed October 3, 2024, https://naprotechnology.com/.

85–86 "In the Old Testament, the concept of flourishing is best described by the Hebrew word *shalom*": Anne Bradley, "You Are Called to Bring About Flourishing," Institute for Faith, Work & Economics, September 18, 2018, https://tifwe.org/you-are-called-to-bring-about-flourishing/.

86 *Shalom* functions in three main ways in the Old Testament: Jonathan T. Pennington, "A Biblical Theology of Human Flourishing," Institute for Faith, Work &

Economics, March 4, 2015, https://tifwe.org/wp-content/uploads/2015/03/A-Biblical-Theology-of-Human-Flourishing-Pennington.pdf. The quote I use is footnoted by Pennington as follows: "This particular breakdown, including the estimates of percentage of usage, comes from John Durham, as summarized in [Perry] Yoder."

89 **"According to the HFEA, in 2017 the simple live birth rate for IVF was 26.4%":** "What is NeoFertility?" NeoFertility, accessed October 3, 2024, https://neofertility.ie/what-is-neo-fertility/.

89 **80 percent of couples with previous miscarriages had successful pregnancies:** "What Can Neo Treat?" NeoFertility, accessed October 3, 2024, https://neofertility.ie/what-can-neo-treat/.

89 **"The lowest AMH blood result we have achieved success with":** "What Can Neo Treat?"

90 **Endometriotic lesions are excised:** "What Can Neo Treat?"

90 **A patient had three successful pregnancies even though she had PCOS:** "Claire and Dave, 3 Healthy Neo Babies." NeoFertility website, July 17, 2020, https://neofertility.ie/neo_story/claire-and-dave-3-healthy-neo-babies/.

91–92 **"An approach to reproductive medicine that uses medical and surgical techniques":** "RRM Shows New Hope for Couples After Failed IVF," International Institute for Restorative Reproductive Medicine, September 1, 2018, https://iirrm.org/hope-after-ivf-rrm/.

92 **The International Institute for Restorative Reproductive Medicine (IIRRM) is based in London and has board member physicians from around the world:** "Board of Trustees," International Institute for Restorative Reproductive Medicine," https://iirrm.org/board-of-trustees/.

92 **The IIRRM's website provides links to like-minded organizations in the United States, Europe, Australia, and Africa:** "Useful Links," International Institute for Restorative Reproductive Medicine, accessed October 3, 2024, https://iirrm.org/useful-links/.

93 **"101 patients met the study criteria, among which 74 had a subsequent live birth":** Phil C. Boyle et al., "Healthy Singleton Pregnancies from Restorative Reproductive Medicine (RRM) After Failed IVF," *Frontiers in Medicine* 5 (July 2018), https://www.frontiersin.org/articles/10.3389/fmed.2018.00210/full.

94 "When we adopted my sons": Brianna Heldt, "What is Love?," Brianna Heldt (website), accessed June 12, 2021, http://www.briannaheldt.com/2014/11/21/what-is-love / (site discontinued).

CHAPTER 13

102 "In Christ alone my hope is found": Stuart Townend and Keith Getty, "In Christ Alone," Stuart Townend (website), accessed October 3, 2024, https://www.stuarttownend.co.uk/song/in-christ-alone/.

102–103 "What is an idol?" John Piper, "What is Idolatry? Interview with John Piper," Desiring God, August 19, 2014, https://www.desiringgod.org/interviews/what-is-idolatry.

107 "O Jesus, I surrender myself to you; take care of everything!": Taylor Tripodi, "Want a Deeper Surrender? Let It Go with This Novena," Ascension Press, August 1, 2019, https://media.ascensionpress.com/2019/08/01/want-a-deeper-surrender-let-it-go-with-this-novena/.

108 "The secret is *Christ* in *me*, not me in a different set of circumstances": Elisabeth Elliot, *Keep a Quiet Heart* (Grand Rapids, MI: Revell, 2021), 20.

108 "The deepest things that I have learned in my own life": "About Elisabeth Elliot," Elisabeth Elliot Foundation, accessed October 3, 2024, https://elisabethelliot.org/about/.

111 "When peace like a river attendeth my way": The hymn quote plus details of Spafford's life taken from "Story Behind the Song: It Is Well with My Soul," *St. Augustine Record*, October 16, 2014, https://www.staugustine.com/article/20141016/lifestyle/310169936.

APPENDIX I

122–123 "The only option that honors the rights of frozen children is not listed on the ASRM": Katy Faust, "Why Embryo Adoption Damages Children's Rights," Them Before Us, December 5, 2019, https://thembeforeus.com/why-embryo-adoption-damages-childrens-rights/.

123 Loeb wants full custody to bring them to term: Cassy Fiano-Chesser, "Sofia Vergara Wins Bid to Decide Fate of Frozen Embryos with Ex-Fiancé Nick Loeb," Live Action News, March 5, 2021, https://www.liveaction.org/news/sofia-vergara-decide-fate-frozen-embryos-loeb/; Nick Loeb, "Sofía Vergara's Ex-Fiancé: Our Frozen Embryos Have a Right to Live," *New York Times*, April 29, 2015, https://www.nytimes.com/2015/04/30/opinion/sofiavergaras-ex-fiance-our-frozen-embryos-have-a-right-to-live.html.